L E A N

&

M E A N

THE NO HASSLE, LIFE-EXTENDING
WEIGHT LOSS PROGRAM FOR MEN

BY MORTON H. SHAEVITZ, PH.D.

G. P. PUTNAM'S SONS
New York

L E A N
&
M E A N

To my sons, Jonathon and Geoffrey,
and my daughters, Erica and Marejka.

G. P. Putnam's Sons
Publishers Since 1838
200 Madison Avenue
New York, NY 10016

The reader is advised to consult with a physician before beginning the program
presented in this book or any other new regimen of diet and exercise.

Responsibility for any adverse effects or unforeseen consequences resulting from
the use of any information contained herein is expressly disclaimed.

Library of Congress Cataloging-in-Publication Data

Shaevitz, Morton H.
Lean and mean : the no hassle, life-extending, weight loss program
for men / by Morton H. Shaevitz.
p.   cm.
Includes bibliographical references.
ISBN 0-399-13803-X (alk. paper)
1. Reducing.   2. Men—Health and hygiene.   I. Title.
RM222.2.S46   1993   92-32691 CIP
613.2'5'081—dc20

Printed in the United States of America

1   2   3   4   5   6   7   8   9   10

This book is printed on acid-free paper.
∞

Part I

THE SCIENCE

OF

WEIGHT

CONTROL

INTRODUCTION

At the age of twenty, I was a junior at the University of California at Los Angeles (UCLA), was 5′10″ tall, and weighed approximately 270 pounds. I'd been overweight all of my life and had been on almost every kind of diet devised by man or doctor, had been given shots and pills, supported, confronted, and cajoled.

That summer, I moved to a fraternity house with a friend, who weighed about 220 pounds. The fraternity house didn't serve meals, and we didn't have much money, so we decided to lose weight together.

We had cereal and milk for breakfast, would make a large salad with low-calorie dressing and water-packed tuna for lunch, and would go out to dinner at a local restaurant and order the cheapest meal on the menu.

The fraternity house had a swimming pool, and I began swimming, first for about twenty to twenty-five minutes a day and finally as much as an hour a day by the end of the summer. I also walked back and forth to campus (even though I had a car and used to drive) and played intramural sports, like volleyball, flag football, and basketball.

By the time the summer was over, I had lost about sixty pounds and my roommate had lost forty. I continued losing weight over retyped many drafts of this book and put up with my tendency never to be satisfied with a good-natured smile, and to Christy Haven, who was always there when she was needed.

Dr. Howard Hunt, former chairman of the Department of Physical Education of UCSD and now president of the Life Management Group, was very helpful in providing information that appears in the chapter on exercise.

I want to thank my good friends, Dr. Stephen and Susan Polis Schutz, for their many suggestions and sharing of expertise. No two people better exemplify the true meaning of friendship than Sue and Steve.

Finally, thanks to my friends and colleagues at Scripps Clinic and Research Foundation. Scripps is that rare health care organization that offers the opportunity to match research interests with clinical reality. I am grateful to have had the opportunity to work with thousands of overweight men (and women) who have shared their stories, triumphs, and frustrations with me.

To protect the privacy of the people I've worked with, names, occupations, and identifying details have been added, deleted, or changed when illustrative material, anecdotes, or a case study is presented.

August 1992

CONTENTS

the following year and got down to about 155 pounds by the time I graduated.

Since then, my weight has ranged between 155 and 170, but I work at it every single day.

Weight loss and obesity have not always been professional concerns of mine. Initially, my primary career orientation was college student mental health. After completing my Ph.D. in clinical psychology at UCLA, I went on to the University of Michigan, where I was an Assistant Professor of Psychology and eventually became the Associate Director of Counseling Services.

I came to the University of California in San Diego (UCSD) as the new Director of Counseling and Psychological Services and Assistant (now Associate) Clinical Professor of Psychiatry in the medical school. A colleague who was putting together a course on nutrition and weight loss in the Adult Education Division of UCSD and knew about my personal weight history asked me to give a talk on "The Psychology of Obesity."

"But I don't know anything about that," I told her.

"Neither does anyone else," she countered. "But you have six months to prepare and there is a $150 honorarium."

Given my meager salary at that time, I think the honorarium was what persuaded me to accept her offer.

THE MYTHS AND THE REALITIES

Over the next six months I did an extensive review of both the scientific literature and what was appearing in the popular press. I found that in the 70s there were a series of myths about obesity including:

1. That it was a symptom of a major underlying psychological disorder.

2. That it was a sign of poor character or lack of will power or discipline.
3. That it was a medical problem best treated by pharmacological intervention (i.e., diet pills).
4. That it was due to a lack of information best treated by finding the "right diet."
5. That it was due to low thyroid or another type of metabolic disorder.

Each one of those myths has been shown to be incorrect. Today we know that:

1. As a group, overweight people are no more psychologically disturbed than people of normal weight. Actually, when overweight people with abnormal psychological test profiles *lose* weight their psychological tests typically become more normal. It is likely that in most cases, being overweight leads to psychological problems, rather than psychological problems causing obesity.

2. Most overweight people are hardworking, responsible, and productive. They are simply overweight, not personally flawed.

3. The widely prescribed amphetamines of the 1970s were found to be addictive and are no longer used for weight control. While the quest for the "magic pill" continues, it is widely accepted that if medication is used to lose weight, it must be used forever: you stop taking the pills, the weight returns.

4. Diets don't work. All diets are short-term changes in eating behavior to achieve weight loss. When people go on a diet, they are just waiting for the diet to end so they can go back to eating "normally"—which means how they ate before they started dieting. And guess what? The weight returns.

5. Only a minuscule number of overweight people have any type of underlying metabolic disorder. Obesity is a result of over-

nutrition, under activity, and influenced, to some degree, by hereditary factors.

When I gave that first weight-loss talk, I discussed those myths and also talked about stress, bingeing, and eating when you're bored or worried. I also spoke about alcohol, and traveling, and restaurant eating, and eating at cocktail parties and happy hours.

There were more than 300 people in the audience that day. Most of them were overweight. The next morning my office phone began ringing off the hook. Many of the callers had attended the class and wanted to see me professionally for weight loss. A number of the callers were men. Gradually, I developed a specialty in the treatment of obesity and also began doing research in the area.

For the past twelve years I have been at Scripps Clinic and Research Foundation, where I was the Associate Director of Weight Loss Programs and am currently the Director of Eating Disorders Programs. In these capacities I have worked with thousands of overweight women and men.

SO WRITE A BOOK

Over the years many of the men I worked with successfully have suggested that I write a book about weight control and health for men. They thought that information from a male perspective would be welcomed and that I should share my ideas more broadly.

So I decided that's what I'd do—I'd write a health-enhancement and weight-loss book for men.

I'd put in it the years of experience that I've had in helping men lose weight and keep it off. And I'd do it in a way that took into account how men are living their lives in the 90s—they're busy, stressed, traveling, eating out, they don't have enough time to exercise, and are worried about their health and weight.

When I began talking about this idea, women said that there should be a chapter for them. They said it was frustrating to live with an overweight man that they wanted to help but didn't know what to do or say. Mostly, they were worried about their husbands or boyfriends (or fathers, or sons, or brothers, or even colleagues) getting ill or dying prematurely. Many reported that:

- If they brought the subject up, they were accused of nagging.
- If they ignored the subject, they were accused of not being supportive.
- If they cooked "healthy meals," their men complained about "not wanting to live on alfalfa sprouts and tofu."
- If they prepared regular meals (usually what their men liked), these men would say, "How do you expect me to lose weight when you serve me *this* kind of food?"

Therefore, I have written a special chapter entitled "For the Women Who Love Them."

Most of the men who read this book have been successful at school, and in their careers, and in their relationships. The reason they've not succeeded in losing weight is that they simply *didn't know what to do.*

I want it to be different for you. I guarantee you that if you read this book and follow my recommendations not only will you lose weight but you'll look better, you'll feel better, you'll be happier, and you may live longer!

YOU CAN DO IT.

Acknowledgments

Over the years many men—and the women who love them—have encouraged me to write this book, but it wasn't until the summer of 1990 that the possibility became a reality. During some brisk morning walks while we were at the Stanford Sierra Camp, my son Jonathon literally got me off my duff when he said, "Well, Dad, why don't you just do it!" Since that time Jonathon has been a continual source of information, support, and feedback.

Throughout the writing process my wife, Marjorie, has always been there with honest and helpful comments. Her expertise about women and gender differences is reflected in the chapter "For the Women Who Love Them," and in many other parts of the book.

I want to thank my agent, Margret McBride, and her staff, Winifred, Susan, and Kelly, for their persistence and excitement about this project. I appreciate all of your efforts, especially for introducing me to the wonderful people at Putnam. And speaking of my publisher, my editors, Rena Wolner and Chris Pepe, have been an author's dream . . . enthusiastic, helpful, available, and always positive in their feedback.

A special thanks goes to Nancy Wilson, who patiently typed and

CHAPTER 1

THE LEAN & MEAN APPROACH

Lean & Mean is a program for men who want to look better, feel better, get healthier, live longer, and lose weight.

Lean & Mean is not a deprivation program. It's a man's book, designed for men who travel for business and pleasure, go to restaurants and enjoy eating out, attend dinner parties, go to business luncheons, and in general lead full lives in all respects. It's for men who don't like how they look or feel, know that being overweight is unhealthy, and want to do something about it now!

In this book, I'll describe the physics of food, show you how you can enjoy eating, and actually eat more while losing weight and getting healthy. I'll present a program of exercise involving three steps to fitness that any man can follow and show you that you don't have to change your life in order to have your life change— for the *better.*

So if you're a man who's between twenty-five and seventy-five pounds overweight, and would like to lose weight and keep it off for the rest of your life, Lean & Mean is for you.

WHAT'S HAPPENING TODAY

According to the 1988 National Center for Health Statistics Report, more than 25 million American men are clinically obese, i.e., they are at least 20% above their ideal body weight. Surprisingly, more *men* (25.9%) than *women* (22.3%) are obese.

Another 10 to 15 million men are simply heavier than they'd like to be and would like to feel better, look better, and lose some weight. They're not quite fitting into their 32- or 34-inch pants, feel more fatigued than they'd like to, and they may have even noticed some decrease in their sexual interest.

Men who earn more than $50,000 annually are more than twice as likely to be obese than women who earn more than $50,000 annually (25.9% vs. 12.7%). Men with more than twelve years of education are almost twice as likely to be obese than women with more than twelve years of education (23.5% vs. 14.8%). Thus, the more a man earns and the more education a man has, the more likely he is to be obese.

Moreover, male-pattern obesity (fat carried between the nipples and the navel) is vastly more dangerous than female-pattern obesity (fat carried between the navel and the knees) and is an independent risk factor for the development of cardiovascular disease and diabetes. Obesity is also linked to the development of hypertension, stroke, gallbladder disease, sleep apnea, musculoskeletal problems, and certain forms of cancer.

Aside from smoking, obesity, hypertension and elevated cholesterol are *the* major factors associated with coronary heart disease, the leading killer of men in the United States. Although it is now known that the rate of cardiovascular disease for women parallels that for men, it is generally accepted that men have their heart attacks approximately ten years sooner than women. By age sixty, one in five men have suffered a heart attack as compared to one in seventeen women. *Fat men die young.*

But now the good news. New research indicates that the effects of even modest weight loss in men with obesity-related medical conditions are significant. In fact, losing 10% of body weight or less will lead to substantial improvement in those individuals who have high blood pressure, adult-onset diabetes, and cardiovascular disease, and will increase longevity. Of course you need to keep the weight off, since weight cycling can actually be worse than no weight loss at all. *Losing weight and keeping it off will prolong your life.*

WHY WORRY?

Until recently, a man who was overweight may not have worried about it. Being overweight did not significantly affect his ability to get hired, receive promotions, meet and date attractive women, or be sexually active. While he knew that being "heavy" was not desirable, after having tried a few crash diets and failing, he would tend to minimize the consequences of his flab and get on with his life with an "oh, what the hell" attitude.

But things are changing. Men are now worried. They know that being overweight and eating a high-fat diet is a major risk factor for cardiovascular disease, diabetes, gallbladder disease, musculoskeletal problems (including lower back pain, sprained ankles, and twisted knees), and certain types of cancer. And now a new dimension has been added. Men are beginning to pay many of the social and interpersonal prices associated with being overweight that have, heretofore, affected only women. They now know that appearance is becoming a factor in career advancement, and that the dating scene is also changing.

THE TRUTH ABOUT OVERWEIGHT MEN

The truth is that men hate being overweight. The thousands of overweight men that I have seen in my professional practice:

- **Hated how they looked** (but wouldn't admit it).
- **Felt tired much of the time** (but attributed it to working too hard).
- **Were often depressed about their weight** (but never told anyone).

- **Worried that their being overweight might affect their chances for promotions** (but denied that they were worried).
- **Knew they risked developing or had already developed major medical problems as a result of their weight** (but couldn't conceive that anything serious like a heart attack would ever happen to them).
- **Reported not feeling sexual** (but often blamed their partners).
- **Reported not being sexual, even if they were in a relationship with a willing partner** (but talked of fatigue, or not having enough time, or hectic lifestyles, or, or, or, or).

Most of them understood that being overweight was a health hazard. Many stated that it was affecting them both personally and professionally. When I asked them why they hadn't gotten any help before, most said that they had tried, but there just didn't seem to be anything available to them that made any sense.

They had tried powdered meals or fasting and lost weight, but then gained it all back again. They had been urged to lose weight by their physicians, had been given a thousand-calorie diet and advised to exercise. However, these recommendations were difficult to put into practice.

If they had wives or girlfriends who were trying to lose weight, they would pick up *their* books, but they didn't help very much. These books didn't tell them what to do when they were trying to get a report done at 2:00 in the morning, writing with one hand and eating potato chips with the other, how to handle lunch at an Italian restaurant, and a cocktail party at 7:00 p.m. followed by dinner with a client.

They had tried to get involved in exercise programs, but found that the expectations of their twenty-year-old instructors with 5% body fat were unrealistic and confusing. Most men that I see don't have the time to spend hours in health clubs or gyms. They just want to know what they must do to lose weight, stay healthy, and look good.

GETTING HELP

But when men look for help, it's not easily available. Weight-loss books are written with women readers in mind. Often half of the pages are devoted to calories, complicated "exchange" food plans, low-calorie shopping and cooking, and massive numbers of low-fat, high-fiber, low-cholesterol, low-salt recipes including how food should "look" on the plate. Since most men eat two or even three meals "out" (and rarely shop or cook), men tell me that this kind of information is irrelevant and boring.

Almost every woman's magazine—*Cosmo, Self, Vogue, Good Housekeeping, McCall's, Redbook, Glamour, Vanity Fair*, or even *Seventeen*—has at least one article about weight loss in every issue. The magazines men read—*Fortune, Business Week, Forbes, Esquire, GQ, Sports Illustrated*, or even *Playboy*—rarely, if ever, have articles about weight control, nutrition, food, or healthy living.

Consequently, most men, overweight or not, are truly ignorant about these topics. There is a dearth of information about obesity, health, and weight loss available to men. And that's what this book is all about.

To help you understand more about Lean & Mean, let me tell you about Fred.

When I got the message that Fred had called my office, I assumed that his reason for calling was social, since we had run into one another in a restaurant a few nights ago. What I discovered was that he had just seen an ad about a weight-loss program that I had been conducting at Scripps Clinic and Research Foundation for the past ten years and wanted to know if it made sense for him to enroll.

After hearing about his weight, which involved gaining and losing the same thirty pounds over a twenty-year period, I told him I certainly thought it would make some sense. He also confided that he was on his tenth day of a "total fast." This was the primary method that he had used to lose weight in the past few years, and he asked what I thought. I told him fasting is a terrible way to lose weight, that "total fasting" is life threatening, and that even "modified fasting" programs under medical supervision had a poor history in terms of weight regain.

Fred asked if it would be possible to see me individually as well as attend my program, and I agreed. When Fred came in, he described his current lifestyle. He's in his mid-forties and has been single for the last seven years. He has a very active social life, which includes going out to dinner with colleagues or women friends at least four nights a week.

He travels for business an average of one week out of every four. He starts his work day at 7:00 in the morning, frequently doesn't finish until 8:00 at night, and is usually feeling stressed, tired and hungry by then. If he doesn't go out to dinner, he'll pick up some Chinese food or a pizza on the way home and eat while watching television. After dinner, he often snacks on potato chips or crackers and cheese while reading or watching television, and then falls asleep.

When I asked him what he did for exercise, Fred said that he liked to play racquetball but due to his schedule and the difficulties in finding a partner, he only managed to get a game up once or twice a week. While he was in high school and his first couple of years at college, he had been into athletics, worked out fairly regularly, and didn't have a weight problem.

After graduating college, he took his first job and was married at twenty-four. During the first few years of marriage he gained forty pounds. He began dieting and was fairly successful the first few times, but it became harder to diet as the years progressed.

Then somebody suggested fasting and that worked out fine for him, because it was easier to not eat anything than to diet. Later he consulted a physician, who suggested that Fred use one of the powdered supplements mixed with water. He told Fred that this was a much safer way to fast than eating nothing.

Fred sometimes uses the supplement and sometimes he doesn't. When he loses weight by fasting, it generally takes him less than six months to gain back all the weight he lost. Fred still occasionally tries to lose weight by conventional "dieting," but finds that counting calories just doesn't work.

Sometimes he picks up a weight-loss book or reads an article about losing weight in an airline magazine. None of the recommendations in the articles or books he reads seems relevant to how he lives his business and personal life. He doesn't have the time or interest to cook for himself and nothing that he's read has helped him to deal with his tendency to eat late at night, particularly when he was working on a proposal or was worried about a project that wasn't going well. That's why he was coming to see me.

Fred's situation is pretty similar to what I hear from most men who have weight problems.

- They are living exceedingly complicated lives.
- They travel extensively.
- Most of them have coffee and a doughnut, or if they're trying to be "healthy," a bran muffin (read "fat sponge") for breakfast, go out for lunch every day, and go out for dinner a few nights a week.
- They'd like to exercise but often don't.
- They tend to be evening and late-night eaters and drinkers.
- They've found that most conventional diet programs are not compatible with their personal and professional lifestyle.
- They often gravitate toward simple solutions like fasting or liquid meal substitutes.
- They're becoming more concerned about the health consequences of their being overweight (particularly men over forty), and/or are concerned that being overweight makes them look and feel less attractive.

Let me tell you a few more things about them:

- Most of the men that I talk to are impatient and want fast results.
- Given a choice, they want an approach that is straightforward and simple, rather than convoluted and confusing.

- They have little interest in counting calories or grams of fat or food exchange programs, and their eyes glaze over when somebody begins to talk about "the nutritional needs of the average American man."
- Those men who live alone cook only to survive or show off—one man told me that if not for take-out Chinese food, pizza, and microwave ovens, he might starve to death.
- Those men who are married or live with a woman usually eat what she prepares (good, bad, or indifferent!).

If any of this sounds like you, then you're probably going to find this book interesting and useful.

Now let me tell you what happened to Fred. He did attend my program and we met half a dozen times. He followed almost all the suggestions that I made, lost about thirty pounds over a four-month period, and more than a year later was still maintaining his weight.

- His social life is as full as ever—except that he goes to better restaurants. He reports that since he's lost weight, the quality of his social life is much improved.
- He still travels extensively but finds that traveling causes him fewer problems than it used to as a result of following my recommendations about flying and traveling. His life is still very hectic, and at times frantic, but food is no longer his primary way of dealing with stress.
- He was one of the many men who read this book while it was in draft form and made recommendations to make it even easier to use.

I know that if you follow my suggestions, you can be as successful as Fred. After you've finished reading this book, let me know how it changed your life.

CHAPTER 2

THE ONE, TWO, THREE, FOUR

OF WEIGHT LOSS

Losing weight is easy. Keeping the weight off is difficult. Almost everybody has lost weight in the past. Almost nobody knows how to keep from gaining it back.

Losing weight by not eating or eating only one type of food sounds very appealing because it's so simple. If you do lose weight this way you may be initially successful, but I guarantee you'll gain it all back. In order to lose weight, and to keep it off for the rest of your life, you need to make FOUR (but only four) major changes:

1. SIGNIFICANTLY DECREASE THE AMOUNT OF FAT THAT YOU EAT.
2. EXERCISE 45 MINUTES TO AN HOUR FIVE TO SIX DAYS A WEEK WHILE YOU'RE LOSING WEIGHT. Exercise 30–45 minutes a day four to five days a week to maintain your weight. (What you do and how hard you do it will vary based upon your age, fitness level, and health status, but I guarantee that you won't have to run marathons or out-powerlift Arnold Schwarzenegger.)

3. DRINK NO ALCOHOL WHILE YOU'RE LOSING WEIGHT. HAVE NO MORE THAN TWO DRINKS A DAY FROM THEN ON AND DON'T DRINK ALCOHOL EVERY DAY. (You can deviate from these guidelines on special occasions such as: doubling your net worth; getting the big promotion; finally buying your Porsche Carrera 4 Cabriolet; being upgraded from coach to first class when flying to Australia, Hong Kong, Tokyo, or Zurich; or getting a $5,000 rebate after your IRS audit.)

4. LEARN TO DO THINGS OTHER THAN EAT WHEN YOU'RE FEELING BORED, STRESSED, LOW, SEXUALLY FRUSTRATED, ANGRY, UNDER PRESSURE, OR OTHERWISE UPSET.

You don't have to be *perfect*, but you do have to be *consistent*. As a general guideline, if you are 80% compliant 80% of the time and don't totally foul up the other 20%, you can probably lose weight and maintain that weight loss for the rest of your life.

RATIONALE

Now let's take a look at why this approach works. To begin with, you need approximately twelve calories per pound of body weight every single day to just maintain your weight. For example, a 200-pound man who does not exercise needs approximately 2,400 calories a day. If you can eliminate 500 or 600 calories per day by decreasing your fat intake and limiting alcohol, and use up an additional 300 or 400 calories a day exercising, you will create a deficit of 1,000 calories per day.

In 7 days you will have created a deficit of 7,000 calories. Since a pound of fat is approximately 3,500 calories, by making these changes, you can lose about two pounds of fat per week. (See Figure I)

While these changes *seem* simple, making them is difficult. Here's why:

1. Decreasing Fats

We like foods that are high in fats, and fat comes in very tasty packages. For example, here are some favorite foods, their approximate calorie count, and what percent of calories comes from fat:

- Prime Rib (100 calories per ounce, 60% of the calories from fat);
- Salad dressings (250 calories per serving, 90% of the calories from fat);
- Cheese (100 calories per ounce, 70% of the calories from fat);
- Premium ice cream (100 calories per ounce, 75% of the calories from fat);
- Avocado dip (75 calories per tablespoon, 80% of the calories from fat);
- And the potato chips or corn chips that we put into that dip (160 calories per ounce, 60% of the calories from fat).

Lean & Mean shows you how to give up fats without giving up satisfaction. In the appendix on page 155 you will find the calorie count and fat percentages of most of the foods you eat on an everyday basis.

2. Exercising Regularly

While everybody knows they *should* exercise regularly, very few men *do* exercise regularly. The reason is a combination of misinformation about what kind of exercise to do, lethargy, overload, time pressure, and boredom. Most men live very complicated

FIGURE I

BEFORE	AFTER
Lean & Mean	Lean & Mean

1. CALORIES IN FROM FOODS AND ALCOHOL: 2,400

2. CALORIES OUT VIA USUAL ACTIVITIES $12 \times 200 = 2,400$

3. CALORIES OUT VIA EXERCISE: 0

4. TOTAL CALORIES OUT: $2,400 + 0 = 2,400$

5. CALORIES IN − CALORIES OUT: $2,400 − 2,400 =$ 0/DAY DEFICIT

6. DEFICIT PER WEEK: $7 \times 0 = 0$

7. WEIGHT LOSS PER WEEK: DEFICIT PER WEEK

3,500 (CALORIES IN 1 LB. FAT)
$$\frac{0}{3,500} = 0 \text{ lbs/WEEK}$$
WEIGHT LOSS

1. CALORIES IN FROM FOOD AND ALCOHOL: 1,800

2. CALORIES OUT VIA USUAL ACTIVITIES $12 \times 200 = 2,400$

3. CALORIES OUT VIA EXERCISE: 400

4. TOTAL CALORIES OUT: $2,400 + 400 = 2,800$

5. CALORIES IN − CALORIES OUT: $1,800 − 2,800 =$ [1,000]/ DAY DEFICIT

6. DEFICIT PER WEEK: $7 \times 1,000 = 7,000$

7. WEIGHT LOSS PER WEEK: DEFICIT PER WEEK

3,500 (CALORIES IN 1 LB. FAT)
$$\frac{7,000}{3,500} = 2 \text{ lbs/WEEK}$$
WEIGHT LOSS

lives, have too many things to do, and not enough time to do them. But,

- Exercise won't happen if you try to *find* the time.
- Exercise can only happen if you *plan* the time.

Lean & Mean will teach you what kinds of exercise are most effective for weight loss and how to assure that you'll do them.

3. Limiting Alcohol

If you don't drink alcohol, skip this section. If you do drink alcohol, you need to read this section. Alcohol is an easy way to take in calories, since only 1½ oz. of 80 proof liquor is 120 calories.

Alcohol affects food intake by decreasing your blood sugar level, which causes you to feel hungry. New research indicates that alcohol makes it more difficult to metabolize fat. Alcohol also affects your judgment and makes it seem all right to eat another few pieces of bread and butter and order chocolate cheesecake for dessert.

To make things simple, I suggest that you don't drink any alcohol at all while you're trying to lose weight. After you've lost all the weight you want, *Lean & Mean* will show you how to include alcohol in your life (if you wish) while maintaining your weight loss.

4. Controlling Stress Eating

If you were to take five minutes and write down each thing you ate over the last 24 hours and next to each entry write down *why* you ate what you did, you would probably find that:

- You were biologically hungry (growly stomach, headachy, or dizzy) less than half the time you ate.
- You did some of your eating because of how good the food

looked, smelled, or tasted (even when you were no longer hungry).

- You did some of your eating because you were taking a coffee break and there was a box of doughnuts in the coffee room (even though you weren't hungry), were at a cocktail party where food was served (even though you weren't hungry), or went to happy hour at a place that had free "snacks" (even though you weren't hungry).

- You did some of your eating because you were feeling stressed, bored, angry, pressured, rejected, or even mildly depressed (even though you weren't hungry).

Lean & Mean will help you understand *why you eat and how to change eating behavior that is harmful.*

Remember, in order to lose weight and maintain that weight loss, you only have to make these four changes. Also remember that consistency is the key!

WHY DECREASE FATS

Fats have more than twice the number of calories than any other source of food (nine calories/gram as opposed to four calories/gram for carbohydrates and protein). A high-fat diet is also linked with elevated cholesterol levels, cardiovascular disease, and other health problems. Reducing fats is the simplest way to decrease your calorie intake, lose weight, and enhance your health status.

WHY EXERCISE

The effects of exercise are multidimensional and appear to be much more complicated than we had first thought. Not only do calories continue to be used during the exercise period, but more calories are used for some time after the exercise period has ended (what is known as the "post-exercise effect"). Another thing that happens when you exercise is a decrease in stress levels and a feeling of well-being. Finally, moderate exercise decreases appetite.

You don't have to do anything as dramatic as train for a marathon to get the benefits of exercise. Walking briskly for forty-five minutes a day is sufficient during the weight-loss phase. You *do* have to exercise consistently. And unless you have major medical or musculoskeletal problems, anyone can exercise.

WHY LIMIT ALCOHOL

Alcohol is one of the three legal drugs frequently used to affect mood. (Caffeine and nicotine are the other two.) Alcohol is a potent source of calories. Having a mixed drink before dinner and two glasses of wine with dinner can easily add 500 calories to your total intake. Alcohol is a central nervous system depressant and impairs judgment. After the third glass of wine, you're much more likely to order the prime rib rather than broiled swordfish and have blue cheese dressing on your salad, and put butter, sour cream, and bacon bits on your baked potato. Alcohol inhibits fat metabolism.

Not drinking alcohol during weight loss will increase your weight-loss rate. Controlled drinking from then on will help you keep the weight off and lead to better overall health.

WHY CONTROL STRESS EATING

Learning how *not* to eat in response to negative emotion is one of the core elements of long-term weight management. We know that all eating is mediated in the part of the brain known as the hypothalamus. We also know that stress eating is not restricted to humans. Mice who previously had eaten their fill will begin eating again when subjected to some mild discomfort and will stop eating when the discomfort ceases. Research on human eating behavior indicates that most instances of uncontrolled and unanticipated eating are associated with feelings of boredom, sadness, or anger. Chapter 7 deals with the issue of stress-induced eating in great depth.

FINALLY

Will the Lean & Mean Program guarantee that you'll get healthier, lose weight and keep the weight off? Yes, so long as you *follow the program.*

- To become a class A tennis player you need to take lessons *and* play a few times a week *and* work on the problems in your game. Just spending a week at a tennis camp is not enough.
- To be a four-handicap golfer you need to work with a pro *and* play regularly *and* go to the driving range. Just taking six lessons is not enough.
- To get healthy, lose weight, and *keep* the weight off for the rest of your life you need follow the Lean & Mean Routine forever.

Deprivation doesn't work. Pills don't work. Will power doesn't work.

LEAN & MEAN WORKS

What I'll be doing in subsequent chapters is to provide you with a structured road map of how to apply these principles as you live your busy life. For the moment, remember the word SAFE as a summary of the Lean & Mean Routine:

- Reduce   **S**tress eating
- Control   **A**lcohol
- Decrease **F**ats
- Increase **E**xercise

CHAPTER 3

THE PHYSICS OF FOOD

A few years ago I was speaking before almost one thousand people on the topic of weight loss. I had just finished a presentation on basic nutrition and asked if there were any questions. One man put up his hand and when I acknowledged him he asked, "Dr. Shaevitz, can you tell me the number of calories there are in anchovies?"

"Anchovies, anchovies," I said, half aloud. "Well let's see, anchovies are a fish but, of course, they're packed in oil. By the way," I said, "why are you asking?"

"Well," replied my questioner, "I'm going out for pizza this evening and I wanted to know whether to order the pizza with the anchovies or without the anchovies."

"You know," I replied, "if you're just going to eat one or two slices of pizza it really doesn't make any difference whether you have them with or without anchovies. And you know," I went on further, "if you are going to eat a whole pizza, the last thing you have to worry about is whether you have anchovies on them."

Overall, I find that many people who talk about nutrition make it too complex. My good friend, Jean Jones, a nutritionist and author of more than twenty books in the area of high-quality eating and healthy cooking, says: "Nutrition is my favorite subject because it's so easy."

34

So now let me tell you everything you need to know about nutrition in order to lose weight while eating more food, increase your health status and keep that weight off for the rest of your life.

There are only three (3) kinds of food in the world and only four (4) sources of calories. The three kinds of food are: fats, proteins, and carbohydrates. The four sources of calories are these three foods plus alcohol.

- Fats have 9 calories per gram,
- Alcohol has 7 calories per gram,
- Protein and carbohydrates have 4 calories per gram.

If you want to lose fat and increase your health, you need to:

FIGURE I

1. *SIGNIFICANTLY DECREASE* THE AMOUNT OF FAT (BOTH ANIMAL AND VEGETABLE) THAT YOU EAT.

2. *SIGNIFICANTLY INCREASE* THE AMOUNT OF COMPLEX CARBOHYDRATES (ANYTHING THAT GROWS AND IS NOT REFINED) THAT YOU CONSUME.

3. *LIMIT* YOUR ALCOHOL INTAKE.

---

1. Decrease Fats

There are two ways to decrease the amount of fat you consume. The first way is obvious, the second, subtle. The first way is to limit the foods that you know are high in fat—butter, margarine, regular salad dressings, mayonnaise, avocados, ice cream, gravy, rich desserts, and fried foods.

The second way is to decrease the portion size of foods that have a high percentage of fat in them—primarily cheeses and animal protein. Between 60% and 90% of the calories in cheese come from fat. By using cheese only to add flavor, you can easily reduce fats from this source.

Animal protein (poultry, shell fish, fish, pork, beef, lamb, and veal) has between 30% and 70% of calories coming from fat. By reducing your portions of animal protein to no more than six ounces per day and by making low-fat choices like fish, poultry, and shellfish, rather than high fat choices like beef, lamb, pork, and veal, you automatically decrease the amount of fat in your diet.

2. Increase Complex Carbohydrates

This is relatively easy to do and allows you to eat a lot of food while still losing weight. While celery and carrots are thought of as being the usual "diet foods," breads, rolls, potatoes, and pastas are all sources of complex carbohydrates and good weight-loss foods if you limit the butter and sauces. You can also feel fairly comfortable eating generous portions of cereals (except granola and the like), fruits, salads (control the dressing), and vegetables (without cheese sauces).

3. Limit Alcohol

For the moment, think of alcoholic beverages as a potent source of calories—ranging from 160 for a large glass of wine to 500 calories for a good size margarita. Don't drink while you're losing weight and limit yourself to only two drinks per day to maintain your weight loss.

OPTIMAL EATING DURING MAINTENANCE

An optimal eating program (after the weight loss phase) will have 60–65% of your calories coming from complex carbohydrates, 20% of your calories coming from protein, and less than 20% of calories coming from fat (the less the better), with a maximum of two drinks per day.

The closer you can get to this ideal, the healthier you will be, the leaner you will be, and the *more food* (by volume) you get to eat. You can eat this way while going to restaurants, eating at other people's homes, eating on airplanes, attending conventions, going to cocktail parties, and living a full life.

You don't have to eat twigs, berries, alfalfa sprouts, or any other kinds of exotica. You just have to make good choices. The other chapters in this book will tell you how to make those choices.

MORE ABOUT CARBOHYDRATES

Carbohydrates can be broken down into two types. There are complex carbohydrates and simple carbohydrates. A complex carbohydrate is anything that grows and *hasn't been* refined—things like fruits, vegetables, grain cereals, whole grain breads. Complex carbohydrates contain fiber and high levels of essential nutrients, including vitamins, minerals, and trace elements.

Take a complex carbohydrate and refine it and you have a simple carbohydrate like sugar, white flour, or corn syrup. By refining a complex carbohydrate, you remove the fiber and essential nutrients and also increase the calorie density. A sugar beet that weighs a pound only contains about 180 calories. A pound of sugar (which is derived from the sugar beet) contains approximately 2,000 calories.

When you make complex carbohydrates simple, you increase calories and take away food value. That's why dietitians recommend that you eat more complex carbohydrates and fewer simple carbohydrates. Of course, there are times that you want something sweet and don't want to eat a sugar beet. In subsequent chapters I'll tell you how to self-indulge responsibly.

MORE ABOUT PROTEIN

There are two types of protein, animal and vegetable. Both sources of protein have four calories per gram, but when you eat animal protein, fat comes along for the ride. Remember, fat has nine calories per gram. The more you eat animal protein, the more fat calories you consume. Obviously, the better option is to choose low-fat proteins like fish, fowl, and shellfish, and limit how much and how often you eat high-fat animal proteins like beef, pork, and lamb.

So why not get all our protein from plants? First, because most of us like the taste of grilled steak, roast chicken, steamed lobster, and broiled swordfish. Second, because while animal proteins contain all twenty-two essential amino acids and are a "complete" protein, plants have only some of the essential amino acids. So we have to be pretty good at eating a variety of plant sources in order to get a complete protein. Those who are vegetarians know how to do this with something called protein complementarity (for example: beans and rice). If you want to get more of your protein from plants, or even consider vegetarianism, read one of the books listed in the Suggested Reading or consult a registered dietitian.

MORE ABOUT FATS

Fat is high in calories, about nine calories per gram. But some fat is worse for you than others. Fat that comes from animal sources (butter, lard, and a well-marbled steak) is saturated fat and contains cholesterol. This is bad fat. Fat that comes from plant sources like olive oil, corn oil, and peanut oil, and has not been hydrogenated, still has the same nine calories per gram. But since it is not saturated, it does not tend to have the same effect on your coronary arteries. These fats are poly-unsaturated and/or mono-unsaturated and are less harmful.

Since most of you are not interested in the biochemistry of lipid metabolism, my general recommendation is to significantly decrease the *total amount* of fat in your diet. That means limiting animal protein to 6 oz. a day, and eating high-fat animal protein like beef, lamb, or pork only once or twice a week. Have all visible fat trimmed and have your food broiled, steamed, or sautéed with minimal butter or margarine, and have all sauces on the side.

Lowering the fats in your diet also means decreasing the use of salad dressings, gravies, pastries, whole milk, and premium ice cream, and most of all, deciding *how* and *when* you want to take your fat. Would you rather have a pat of butter on your roll or some hollandaise sauce on your asparagus, steak as an entrée or crème caramel for dessert? The choice is yours.

MORE ABOUT ALCOHOL

Alcohol is a particularly potent source of calories and, as you will find out when you read the chapter on booze, alcohol also makes it more difficult to control your food intake. Alcohol also makes it more difficult to use fat as fuel. Excess alcohol intake (we're still not quite sure exactly what that means) tends to elevate triglyceride levels and increase blood pressure. Alcohol has recently been linked to oral and liver cancer in proportion to the amount of alcohol consumed. So in addition to making it really hard to lose weight, drinking a lot of alcohol may contribute to the development of other kinds of medical problems.

WHAT ABOUT CAFFEINE, SALT,
AND WATER?

Here the jury is still out. Depending on what you read, caffeine is or is not associated with the development of certain types of cancer, hypertension, cardiovascular disease, and the like. My advice is moderation—no more than two cups of caffeinated coffee per day on the average. Watch out for diet soft drinks with caffeine—they can add to your caffeine load and lead to the jitters.

The issue of salt is a bit more complicated. If you are one of those people who are sensitive to salt in terms of the development of hypertension and have high blood pressure, you may have to reduce your intake for health reasons. If you don't have high blood pressure, it may not make any difference. Only you and your doctor know for sure.

The last issue is water. Many weight-loss programs advocate that you drink six to eight glasses of water per day. My own view is that increasing fluid intake is probably a good thing. It does make you feel full and you won't rust! Rather than a rigid number of glasses per day, try drinking a full glass of water before each meal. This will increase your fluid intake and help you eat more moderately at meals.

Now that you have all the information you need about nutrition, let's move on.

CHAPTER 4

NEVER ORDER A CHEF'S SALAD AND
A DIET COKE FOR LUNCH

In the fall of 1990 I had the honor of being asked to make two presentations at the Sixth International Congress on Obesity that was being held in Kobe, Japan. Since this was my first trip to the Far East, I decided to make a stop in Hong Kong and then visit some friends in Tokyo.

I had always believed that obesity was primarily a problem of the United States and Western Europe. Traditionally, Asians have been thought of as being lean and slender. While the recent research literature has suggested that the problem was becoming international, I was not prepared for what I observed.

In Hong Kong, particularly in the affluent areas, I was struck by the number of overweight adults and adolescents I saw. In Tokyo I was astounded. Not only did there seem to be a fair number of overweight adults, but I was shocked by the number of truly obese children that I observed. When I went on to the meeting in Kobe, all of my observations were confirmed.

It appears as though the Far East is in the midst of an obesity epidemic. Reports from Cambodia, Thailand, Taiwan, and Hong Kong all indicated that obesity was becoming a major problem. The question, of course, was why? My first day in Kobe, when I went to lunch with some Japanese colleagues, I discovered the answer.

One of the things that I do when I travel abroad is to try to eat "local." This often means only going out once or twice to what might be the equivalent of a four-star restaurant and spending more time eating at cafés, restaurants in department stores, or even buying food from street vendors. The International Congress on Obesity was held at a convention center in Kobe. Directly behind the convention center was a series of small restaurants—sit-down and take-out. What I usually did for lunch was to find one of the noodle or rice shops and get a large bowl filled with noodles or rice with a few slivers of fish or chicken and vegetables on top. This is very filling, and, as you now know, is very low in calories because rice and noodles are basically complex carbohydrates.

What were my colleagues from Japan, Taiwan, Cambodia, and Thailand ordering? They were going next door to a fast-food restaurant and getting a double cheeseburger, french fries, a chocolate malt, and an apple turnover.

We ate the same *amount* of food in terms of *volume*, but at every meal they were eating three times the number of calories that I was. Most of those calories were coming from fat. Most of that fat was saturated fat. As I talked with my colleagues at the meeting, it soon became apparent why there was a major obesity problem and related medical problems in the Far East.

The nature of the food supply had changed from being very high in complex carbohydrates (rice, noodles, bean sprouts, etc.) to a more Western diet, which was extremely high in fat. So not only were there fast-food hamburger restaurants now, there was take-out pizza, fried chicken restaurants, or a premium ice-cream store on almost every street corner. While the people had maintained the volume of food they were eating, now they were eating food that was 50–60% fat and, as a consequence, obesity is now becoming a major problem in the Far East. They call it the McDonaldization of the Orient.

In this chapter I'll show you how to lower significantly the percentage of fat that you consume, eat more food, and lose weight. The way to achieve low-fat eating is to:

FIGURE I

1. NEVER ORDER A CHEF'S SALAD AND A DIET COKE FOR LUNCH.

2. OR A LARGE ORANGE JUICE, A BRAN MUFFIN, AND BLACK COFFEE FOR BREAKFAST.

3. OR OYSTERS ROCKEFELLER, SALAD WITH BLUE CHEESE DRESSING, PRIME RIB, BAKED POTATO WITH BUTTER, SOUR CREAM, AND BACON, AND CHEESECAKE FOR DINNER.

Why? Because *eating fat makes you fat.*

And because each of these meals provides you with a relatively small amount of food and an enormously large number of calories for the amount of food being eaten. Most of those calories come from saturated fat, which is particularly bad for you if you're a man. A high-fat diet keeps you fat and will lead to heart disease. (See Figure II A, B, C)

FIGURE II A
TYPICAL LUNCH

Food	Calories	Percentage Calories from Fat	Calories from Fat	Weight of Food
Chef's Salad				
4 oz. Salad	100	0%	0	4 oz.
2 oz. Cheese	200	90%	180	2 oz.
2 oz. Ham	200	80%	160	2 oz.
2 oz. Turkey	100	50%	50	2 oz.
2 oz. Bologna	200	80%	160	4 oz.
Dressing 4 oz.	400	90%	360	4 oz.
Diet Coke	0		0	
	1,200		910	16 oz.

FIGURE II B
TYPICAL BREAKFAST

Food	Calories	Percentage Calories from Fat	Calories from Fat	Weight of Food
Bran Muffin	400	75%	300	4 oz.
Butter (2 Pats)	100	100%	100	1 oz.
Large Orange Juice	150	0%	0	0 oz.
	650		400	5 oz.

FIGURE II C
TYPICAL DINNER

Food	Calories	Percentage Calories from Fat	Calories from Fat	Weight of Food
Oysters Rockefeller	450	80%	360	6 oz.
Salad	50	0%	0	2 oz.
Blue Cheese Dressing	250	90%	225	3 oz.
Prime Rib (8 oz.)	800	60%	480	8 oz.
Baked Potato	150	0%	0	12 oz.
3 Pats Butter	150	100%	150	3 oz.
1 Tbs. Sour Cream	75	80%	60	2 oz.
Cheese Cake	500	90%	450	6 oz.
	2,225		1,725	38 oz.

NOTE: No alcohol, no bread and butter.

So what can you order instead?

Here are some better alternatives.

1. What to Eat for Lunch

1. A sliced turkey sandwich with lettuce, tomatoes, and mustard, or just a dab of mayonnaise, a side of vinegar-based coleslaw, and iced tea.

2. A green salad with dressing on the side; grilled halibut and rice pilaf or a baked potato; a roll and coffee.

3. Wonton soup, shrimp and vegetables, white rice, tea and a fortune cookie.

And if you want something sweet, a nonfat yogurt as you walk back to the office.

2. What to Eat for Breakfast

Start with half a cantaloupe or a bowl of strawberries or sliced bananas. Then you can have toast or an English muffin, or a toasted bagel with a bit of jam or jelly; or a short stack of pancakes or a small waffle (with scant butter and just enough syrup for taste), or a bowl of hot or cold cereal with low or nonfat milk.

3. What to Eat for Dinner

Start with oysters on the half shell, or a shrimp cocktail, or seviche, or onion soup (light on the cheese, please); followed by a green salad with vinaigrette dressing on the side, and a couple wedges of lemon (squeeze the lemon juice on the salad, put a teaspoonful of salad dressing on the salad, and mix); then broiled swordfish or chicken or steamed lobster or crab legs (limit how much drawn butter you use); and finally, raspberries and cappuccino for dessert (or if there is something that's truly wonderful for dessert, split it with your colleagues, wife, or girlfriend).

If you will make these changes (or changes like these) at every meal every day, at the end of a week you will lose between one and two pounds of fat. At the end of a month, you will lose between five and eight pounds of fat. At the end of a year you can have lost *all the weight you want*. You will also have significantly lowered your serum cholesterol level and have slowed or prevented the development of cardiovascular disease.

If you make these changes half the time, you lose half as much weight. If you eat this way only twice a week you will lose two sevenths as much weight.

So without starving, without having to change where you eat or when you eat, and without having to be a real pain to yourself and those around you, you can lose the excess fat that you put on over the last five, ten, or twenty years.

Do you know that if you make these changes you will actually be eating more food than you are currently eating now and lose weight? How can you *eat more* and *weigh less*?

How does this work? Take a look at Figures III A,B,C:

FIGURE III A
USUAL LUNCH

Food	Calories	Percentage Calories from Fat	Calories from Fat	Weight of Food
Chef's Salad				
4 oz. Salad	100	0%	6	4 oz.
2 oz. Cheese	200	90%	180	2 oz.
2 oz. Ham	200	80%	160	2 oz.
2 oz. Turkey	100	50%	50	2 oz.
2 oz. Bologna	100	80%	100	4 oz.
Dressing (4 oz.)	400	90%	360	4 oz.
Diet Coke	0		0	
	1,200		850	16 oz.

LEAN & MEAN LUNCH

Food	Calories	Percentage Calories from Fat	Calories from Fat	Weight of Food
Sliced Chicken Sandwich with Lettuce, Tomato, Mustard	325	20%	65	8 oz.
Coleslaw	75	0%	0	4 oz.
Ice Tea	0	0%	0	
	400			12 oz.
Optional Nonfat Yogurt	150	0%		6 oz.
	550		65	18 oz.

FIGURE III B
USUAL BREAKFAST

Food	Calories	Percentage Calories from Fat	Calories from Fat	Weight of Food
Bran Muffin	400	75%	300	4 oz.
Butter (2 Pats)	100	100%	100	1 oz.
Large Orange Juice	150	0%	0	
	650		400	5 oz.

LEAN & MEAN BREAKFAST

Food	Calories	Percentage Calories from Fat	Calories from Fat	Weight of Food
$^1/_3$ Cantaloupe	75	0%	0	5 oz.
2 Toast, or 1 Bagel, or 1 English Muffin	140	Scant	10	2 oz.
$^1/_2$ Tsp. Jam	75	0%	0	Scant
1 Small Bowl Cereal, Cold	120	Scant	10	$1^1/_2$ oz.
4 oz. Skim Milk	40	0%	0	
	450		20	$8^1/_2$ oz.

FIGURE III C
USUAL DINNER

Food	Calories	Percentage Calories from Fat	Calories from Fat	Weight of Food
Oysters (6) Rockefeller	450	80%	360	6 oz.
Salad	50	0%	0	2 oz.
Blue Cheese Dressing	250	90%	225	3 oz.
Prime Rib (8 oz.)	800	60%	480	8 oz.
Baked Potato	150	0%	0	12 oz.
3 Pats Butter	150	100%	150	2 oz.
1 Tbs. Sour Cream	75	80%	60	2 oz.
Cheese Cake	500	90%	450	6 oz.
	2,225	77%	1,725	37 oz.

NOTE: No alcohol, no bread and butter

LEAN & MEAN DINNER

Food	Calories	Percentage Calories from Fat	Calories from Fat	Weight of Food
Oysters (6) Half shell	60	15%	9	6 oz.
Salad	50	0%	0	2 oz.
Lemon Juice	0	0%	0	
Tsp. Blue Cheese	75	75%	75	1 oz.
Sword Fish (8 oz.)	400	25%	100	8 oz.
Baked Potato	150	0%	0	12 oz.
1/2 Tsp. Sour Cream	50	50%	25	1 oz.
Steamed Vegetables	100	0%		6 oz.
Cappuccino	15	0%		
	950	22%	209	37 oz.

NOTE: No alcohol, no bread and butter

By eliminating most of the calories coming from fat, you are able to eat as much or more food but take in significantly fewer calories. Fat, as you recall, has more than twice the calories of any other food (nine gram/oz. vs. four gram/oz. for protein and carbohydrate). Many of the foods that you eat sound healthy or are thought of as high-protein foods actually contain a lot of fat: commercial bran muffins may contain 400 fat-laden calories, cheddar cheese (the same 100 calories per ounce as premium ice cream with 70% of the calories coming from saturated fat), peanuts (180 calories per ounce with 65% of the calories coming from fat), and prime rib (100 calories per ounce with as many as 80% of the calories coming from fat) are just a few examples.

To make things worse, the body is able to use and store fat efficiently, so 100% of your fat calories are absorbed while perhaps 80–90% of calories from complex carbohydrates and protein are absorbed and utilized.

Thus, by changing the *type of foods* you eat, you will be able to *eat more* food, *lose weight*, and be *healthier.* On the following pages I've listed 100 things that you can do to lower the amount of fat you eat.

DO'S AND DON'TS FOR BREAKFAST

DON'T eat sweet rolls	**DO** eat hard rolls or toast
DON'T eat bran muffins	**DO** eat English muffins
DON'T eat eggs more than 2 times per week	**DO** eat your eggs boiled, poached or fried with minimal butter in a Teflon pan
DON'T put *a pat* of butter on each piece of toast	**DO** use a thin coating of softened butter for flavor (or skip it entirely)
DON'T order hash brown potatoes with your eggs	**DO** order sliced tomatoes with your eggs
DON'T drink whole milk	**DO** drink low-fat or nonfat milk

DON'T pour melted butter on pancakes and waffles

DO use small amounts of syrup or jam and just a bit of melted butter for taste

DON'T put a thick layer of cream cheese on your bagel

DO use a *thin* layer of cream cheese, jelly or whatever on your bagel

DON'T use cream, half-and-half, or commercial creamers in your coffee

DO use low-fat milk in your coffee

DON'T always follow these guidelines

DO have one thing you really love to eat for breakfast once a week

Do's and Don'ts for Lunch

DON'T eat chicken nuggets at fast-food restaurants

DO eat a broiled chicken sandwich

DON'T eat hamburgers with cheese and bacon

DO eat a plain hamburger

DON'T eat french fries with your sandwich

DO eat a salad with your sandwich

DON'T have a milk shake with your meal

DO have iced tea, sparkling water with lemon, a regular or diet soda, or just plain water with your meal

DON'T have a pastry for dessert

DO have a low-fat yogurt or an apple for dessert

DON'T go to fast-food restaurants when you go out for lunch

DO go to delis, coffee shops, and regular restaurants when you go out for lunch

DON'T order soups like Boston clam chowder or cream of chicken soup for lunch

DO order Manhattan clam chowder or onion soup for lunch

DON'T order a regular chef's salad—the cheese, salami, and roast beef are high in fat

DO order a chef's salad with turkey only

DON'T order a crab, shrimp, or lobster salad for lunch—the seafood has been mixed with mayonnaise

DO order a crab, shrimp or lobster Louie—the seafood sits on top of the salad

DON'T allow dressing to be put on any salad

DO order the dressing on the side and use no more than one or two teaspoons and only for moisture and flavor

DON'T order a ham and cheese sandwich—never have your bread grilled

DO order a chicken or lean roast beef sandwich—have your bread toasted if you wish

DON'T order mayonnaise-based side dishes like pasta salad, potato salad, or Waldorf salad

DO order side dishes like green salad, sauerkraut, or vinegar-based coleslaw

DON'T eat lots of crackers with your meal

DO eat *a* roll or *a* slice of bread with your meal

DON'T feel you have to eat all the food you've ordered

DO get used to leaving some food on your plate and feeling satisfied but not stuffed when you've finished

DON'T try to be perfect

DO eat exactly what you want for lunch once a week

Do's and Don'ts for Dinner

DON'T eat things like chips, peanuts, cheese, or crackers before dinner

DO eat things like cold vegetables with salsa or yogurt-based dip before dinner

DON'T eat hors d'oeuvres like rumaki, cocktail hot dogs, or Swedish meatballs

DO eat hors d'oeuvres like shrimp, crab legs, or teriyaki chicken

DON'T order restaurant appetizers like lobster bisque, escargots, or clams casino in a restaurant for appetizers. All are very high in fat.

DO order restaurant appetizers like asparagus with vinaigrette, a steamed artichoke, or mussels in marinara sauce in a restaurant. All are very low in fat.

DON'T eat 80% of your food at dinner and in the evening

DO have no more than 40–50% of your food intake for the day at dinner and in the evening

DON'T eat an 8–16 oz. portion when eating red meat, and skip the vegetables and potato

DO eat no more than 6 oz. of red meat and add a large baked potato or portion of rice or pasta and steamed vegetables

DON'T use a lot of butter or margarine on your baked potato

DO use things like yogurt or salsa on your baked potato, or just enough butter or margarine for moisture on your baked potato

DON'T think that butter is less fattening than margarine

DO know that butter and margarine both contain 45 calories for every pat and *must* be used sparingly

DON'T eat more meat if you want "seconds"

DO eat more pasta, rice, or potato if you want "seconds"

DON'T eat beef, pork, lamb, or veal more than twice a week

DO eat more fish, poultry, shellfish, and pasta

DON'T eat food with lots of cheese

DO add cheese for flavor, but *very* sparingly (cheese is very high in fat)

DON'T order fried rice, sweet and sour pork, spare ribs, or egg rolls in a Chinese restaurant

DO order steamed rice or won-ton soup and vegetable-based entrées in a Chinese restaurant. (Ask them to use very little oil in preparation.)

DON'T eat ice cream more than once a week

DO eat nonfat yogurts or water-based sorbets when you feel like a cold dessert

DON'T order fettucini alfredo, pasta with white clam sauce, or veal parmigiana when you go to an Italian restaurant

DO order pasta fixed with olive oil and a touch of Parmesan cheese or a marinara sauce, chicken piccata, or veal marinara when you go to an Italian restaurant (take only half portions)

DON'T eat guacamole dip, re-fried beans, enchiladas or flour tortillas with chips when you go to a Mexican restaurant

DO eat salsa and cold vegetables, rice, tostadas and corn tortillas when you go to a Mexican restaurant

DON'T follow these guidelines all the time

DO have anything you want for dinner once a week

Do's and Don'ts in General

DON'T eat ice cream or candy at the movies

DO eat popcorn without butter at the movies

DON'T eat nachos, pizza, or corn chips at the ball game

DO bring along some fruit or get popcorn at the ball game

DON'T bring along potato chips, corn chips, candy, or doughnuts when you go on a car trip

DO bring along fresh fruit, cold chicken, veggies, and lots of low-calorie drinks when you go on a car trip

DON'T pick up a pepperoni pizza on the way home from work

DO pick up some broiled chicken on the way home from work

DON'T snack on peanuts

DO snack on fruit

DON'T keep ice cream in the house

DO keep frozen yogurt in the house

DON'T eat those packages of nuts when you fly. They're 90 calories a package—2/3 of the calories coming from fat.

DO wait for the meal and get some juice if you're really feeling hungry

DON'T put cream or half-and-half in your coffee or tea

DO put milk or low-fat milk in your coffee or tea

DON'T eat those little snack bags of chips—they're 180 calories a pop

DO eat baked pretzels—much lower in fat and calories

DON'T spend the evening "grazing" on things like chips, crackers and cheese, and peanuts after dinner

DO plan to have something specific like some fruit with a little low-fat cheese, or a bagel, or a bowl of cereal if you like to eat after dinner

LOW FAT—HIGH HEALTH

Both decreasing the amount of fat in your diet and losing fat from your body lowers your chances of developing serious medical problems. Remember, obesity is an independent risk factor for coronary artery disease, diabetes mellitus, gallbladder disease, hypertension, sleep apnea, and some forms of cancer. Men who carry fat in the abdominal area are at even higher risk for developing cardiovascular disease and having heart attacks. Reducing your weight by losing body fat will significantly increase your health status.

A second but related finding is that people who eat high-fat diets, independent of their degree of obesity, are at increased risk

for developing cardiovascular disease. Saturated fats and cholesterol (which come from animal fat) are the real problem. That's
why the American Heart Association suggests that the percentage
of fat in the the American diet be less than 30%. To reverse
cardiovascular disease, some researchers recommend that less
than 10% of your total intake come from fat. I suggest that 20% be
the upper limit and that you do whatever you can to keep fats
down below that level.

What happens when you decrease your fat intake? Not only
does it lead to weight loss, it also leads to decreased levels of
serum cholesterol, and over a period of time the rate at which you
develop coronary artery disease can be slowed and, some physicians believe, possibly reversed.

Recently, cardiologist Dr. Dean Ornish has reported that his
program of decreased fat, exercise, and stress reduction showed
documented reversal of coronary artery disease. So, a low-fat
eating program will allow you to eat more food, lose weight, and
get healthy.

Now that you have your eating under control, let's move on to
exercise.

CHAPTER 5

THREE STEPS TO FITNESS

A few years ago, I was a speaker on a fourteen-day Mediterranean cruise with the Northern California Pediatric Society. We were on an older ship that had been refurbished, so the exercise facility was down below decks and consisted of two stationary bicycles, a good-sized swimming pool, and a large, carpeted area facing a mirror. Around the perimeter of the room were dumbbells and weights. There was enough room for perhaps half a dozen people to be working out at the same time.

On the first day or two, the exercise room was filled with gasping, out-of-shape bodies. By day four, the crowd had vanished and only the "regulars" were there. I had my routine set—I came down before breakfast, worked out on the stationary bicycle, swam a bit, and used the dumbbells for about fifteen minutes.

One of my companions was a trim-looking nearly bald gentleman, who every day would turn on his mini boom box and do his own movement routine for about forty-five minutes on the carpet in front of the mirror. We began talking, and he confided to me that he was seventy-eight years old. He had been retired for thirteen years. One of the decisions he had made at the time he retired was that he would get up every morning by 7:00, shave, get dressed, and do an hour of physical exercise. I asked him why he had made that deci-sion and he said, "I can't help *getting* old, but I don't have to *be* old."

My friend Rick, whom you'll meet in a future chapter, after a number of years of off-again, on-again exercising not only moved his office to a building that has an exercise club on-site, but has just purchased a stationary bicycle so that if he can't exercise at work, he can exercise at home.

My patient Fred, who you met in chapter 1, checks out every hotel when he's going to a new city to find out the one that has an exercise facility that opens by 6:00 A.M. and stays open until 9:00 P.M. and, except in an emergency, won't go to any other kind of hotel.

Finally, one of my colleagues, an internationally known scientist in cardiovascular disease, and I were talking and he mentioned going to a convention in Dallas. During the time he was there, there were tornadoes and bad weather that made it impossible for anyone to go outside. Unfortunately, the hotel the convention was in didn't have an exercise facility.

"So what did you do?" I asked.

"I walked up and down the stairs for forty-five minutes a day."

"But wasn't that boring?" I said.

He looked at me somewhat quizzically and said, "Sure, but what difference does that make?"

Each of the men I described has decided to make exercise a significant part of his life. Each one has done it in a different way.

If you really want to exercise you can make it happen! My recommendations for exercise are:

FIGURE I

1. IN ORDER TO LOSE A SIGNIFICANT AMOUNT OF BODY FAT, YOU WILL NEED TO EXERCISE 45 MINUTES TO 1 HOUR PER DAY, 5–6 DAYS A WEEK. IN ORDER TO MAINTAIN THAT WEIGHT LOSS YOU WILL NEED TO EXERCISE AT LEAST 30–45 MINUTES A DAY 4–5 DAYS A WEEK FOR THE REST OF YOUR LIFE.

2. 30–45 MINUTES OF EXERCISE SHOULD BE AN AEROBIC ACTIVITY LIKE WALKING, JOGGING, RUNNING, CYCLING, SWIMMING, JAZZERCISE, ETC. A 30–45-MINUTE BRISK WALK IS A PERFECTLY ACCEPTABLE AEROBIC ACTIVITY.

3. FOR THOSE INTERESTED IN MAINTAINING ADEQUATE FLEXIBILITY AND GOOD MUSCLE TONE, APPROXIMATELY 15 MINUTES PER EXERCISE PERIOD NEEDS TO BE DEVOTED TO OTHER ACTIVITIES LIKE *STRETCHING* AND USING *LIGHT WEIGHTS*.

- Don't *think* about exercising
- Don't *worry* about exercising
- Don't *debate* about exercising

As the guys in the ads say—JUST DO IT. And, of course, *always check with your physician before starting any exercise program.*

1. 45–60 Minutes, 5–6 Days a Week During Weight Loss

The most difficult thing about this requirement is finding the time—and, of course, it can't be *found* but must be *created*. In most cases, the best time to exercise is first thing in the morning, because most men will find themselves too tired and too overloaded at the end of the day. When away from home, using the noon hour as an exercise time and then having a light lunch often works out. Many men now have small work-out areas in their home study or bedroom, and an excellent mode of aerobic exercise is using a stationary bicycle (just be sure that you read, listen to music, or watch television so you won't get bored).

2. Aerobic Activity

Whatever aerobic activity you choose, start slowly and increase gradually. The reason most men stop exercising is that they try to do too much too fast. To illustrate what I mean, here's how to start a walking program. To walk, all you need are the right shoes (those designed for walking or jogging) and the right environment. You already know how to walk!

Start with 15–20 minutes per day on a level surface and add 5 minutes per week. Don't worry about speed—concentrate on consistency and endurance. When you have reached forty-five minutes per day, begin walking more briskly. You use almost the same number of calories walking a mile as running a mile. If you can walk a mile in fifteen minutes, that's good. If you can walk a mile in twelve minutes, that's fantastic. If you can walk a mile in less than ten minutes—you're jogging.

3. Flexibility and Toning

For basic flexibility and toning, a flat surface and four pairs of dumbbells, ranging in weight from 5–20 pounds, are all you need. For those interested in becoming more fit or developing greater strength and/or muscle definition, you'll need to work harder and/ or longer. The best way to learn how to stretch and use weights correctly is to consult with an exercise physiologist and/or join a professionally supervised health facility. If these are not readily available, ask your physician or consult one of the books listed in the Suggested Reading section.

a. Why 45–60 Minutes, 5–6 Days a Week During Weight Loss

In order to burn sufficient calories to contribute to your weight loss and allow you to maintain your weight while eating reasonably, you need to exercise longer and more frequently than you'd have to simply to obtain adequate cardiovascular fitness. Another reason is that an hour is a psychologically contained amount of time that men are used to committing.

Finally, when you do exercise for forty-five minutes to an hour, you are likely to get a post-exercise effect, which means that you continue to use more calories for some time after you have stopped exercising. After you've lost your weight, you can decrease your frequency and/or the length of your workout if you want to. Most men continue the 45–60 minutes, 5–6 day routine.

Probably the best reason to exercise this way is that you'll get results and *feel much better!*

b. Why Aerobic Exercise

Until recently the value of exercise and its contribution to weight loss and fitness has been underestimated. The addition of aerobic exercise to a weight-loss program significantly increases the rate of success in both weight loss and weight maintenance. The effect is greater than the actual amount of calorie burnoff, which is contributed by the exercise activity itself.

There are different types of exercise, and each has a different effect. Aerobic exercise literally means *oxygen-using*. The types of exercise that fall into this category are continuous movement activities that use the large muscles of the body and include walking, running, swimming, cycling, using a Stair-master, Jazz-ercise, etc. I recommend that you work up to forty-five minutes per day for the aerobic component. There are benefits to regular aerobic exercise beyond calorie utilization and fitness. Regular aerobic exercise leads to:

1. Increased cardiovascular efficiency, which may slow the development of cardiovascular disease and decrease the likelihood of a heart attack
2. Increased muscle mass
3. Increased fat metabolism
4. Decreased stress
5. Mood stabilization
6. For some people, there's a "post-exercise effect." After you've stopped exercising, you continue to burn more calories per unit of time
7. Decreased appetite
8. Increased adherence to an eating program
9. Possible control of type-2 diabetes without the use of medi-cation when combined with a planned eating program
10. Possible control of mild hypertension without the use of medication when combined with weight loss and salt re-striction.

c. Why Stretching and Weights

There are two other types of exercise—stretching and the use of weights. Stretching will increase flexibility and range of motion and becomes more important as you age. The stretching exercises outlined for you will achieve the goals of allowing full range of motion in all your limbs and torso.

Weight training is the third category of exercise and is designed to increase muscle size and strength. The essential characteristic of weight training is to work a muscle group to exhaustion so that the muscle will grow larger. The results are more size, more definition, and more strength.

FINALLY

Some additional things you might want to know about exercise. The more you weigh, the more calories you use per exercise activity. The reason is very simple. It takes more energy to move a 250-pound person one mile than it does to move a 150-pound person one mile. Thus the benefits of exercise, particularly weight-bearing exercises such as walking, are even greater for big people than for small people.

Exercise also allows you to eat more and maintain your weight, because if you are burning 400 calories per day or 2,400 calories a week by exercising, you can eat an additional 400 calories per day during weight maintenance.

Now that you're eating right and exercising, let's get serious about alcohol.

CHAPTER 6

BOOZE

It is virtually *impossible* to lose weight if you drink a lot. It is very *difficult* to maintain your weight if you drink a lot. Alcohol is a potent source of calories, lowers your blood sugar level, inhibits fat metabolism, and affects your judgment and your ability to make good food choices. The number of calories in a bottle of regular beer (12 oz.), a restaurant-size glass of wine (approximately 6 oz.), or a standard drink without mixer (approximately 1½ oz. of 86 proof whiskey, vodka, gin, scotch, bourbon, tequila) is the same—about 150.

From a health perspective, drinking a lot of alcohol on a regular basis can contribute to developing high blood pressure, raising triglyceride levels, increasing your risk of oral cancer, and may eventually affect your liver so that you will become very, very sick.

Nobody really knows how much alcohol is too much alcohol, but in general, the less often you drink and the less you drink, the better off you are. The following are my recommendations regarding alcohol:

FIGURE I

1. WHILE YOU ARE TRYING TO LOSE WEIGHT, DON'T DRINK ANY ALCOHOL AT ALL.

2. AFTER YOU'RE AT THE WEIGHT YOU WANT TO BE, LIMIT YOURSELF TO TWO DRINKS PER DAY. DON'T DRINK *EVERY* DAY AND DRINK OUT OF *CHOICE* RATHER THAN HABIT.

1. Don't Drink While Losing Weight

Let's keep it simple—don't drink any alcohol while you're losing weight. Don't explain why you're not drinking. Just say, "No thank you." You will likely feel better while not drinking and you'll be less likely to overeat. You may decide to continue your alcohol abstinence when you get to your goal, but if you do want to drink again, then follow my second rule.

2. Most Health Professionals Recommend the Two-Drink Limit

I would also suggest that you make drinking a choice rather than a reflex. Many of my successful patients find that they are able to stick with this guideline by not drinking alone, and only drinking when they are eating and making it part of a social convention. There are many reasons to control alcohol consumption besides health.

Alcohol has a series of effects besides adding unneeded calories. It does tend to lower blood-sugar levels, which can make you feel hungry and eat more. Recent evidence suggests that it makes it more difficult to metabolize fat. Most important, it tends to affect judgment and lead us to do things we might not ordinarily do. The consequence of alcohol consumption is that *cognitive controls* (planning to order the broiled halibut and baked potato) are often affected by alcohol, and so we order food based on our *feelings* (salad with extra blue cheese dressing, fettucini alfredo, and beef Wellington).

The triple trouble of alcohol, then, is that:

1. It's an easy way to get calories;
2. It lowers the blood-sugar level and so increases hunger;

3. And finally, it affects judgment, leading you to make inappropriate food choices.

If you drink less, then drink better quality. Have one or two glasses of a *fine wine* rather than four glasses of an ordinary wine. One of the benefits of decreasing the amount of both the food and alcohol that you consume is that you get to increase quality at approximately the same cost.

Drinking alcohol is a social convention and many people like how alcohol makes them feel. Alcohol is not, as many people think, a stimulant. It is a sedative and a central nervous system depressant. The effect of alcohol is to anesthetize.

If you have any questions about that, recall what happens as you keep drinking. While initially there may be some feelings of exhilaration (having to do with the knocking out of judgment centers), if you continue to drink, you will eventually fall asleep. If you drink too much alcohol in too short a period of time, you can become seriously ill.

If you choose not to drink at all after you've lost your weight, that's fine. If you choose to resume drinking after you've lost weight, remember the two drinks per day limit. And, of course, let's be realistic: for the occasional special event or wonderful celebration—you may choose to bend the rule.

SCIENCE OF ALCOHOL

The essential ingredient in all spirits is alcohol (known as ethanol), created from various ingredients during the fermentation process. Hops and yeast will yield beer. Grapes will yield wine. Potatoes, corn, barley, and cactus will yield vodka, bourbon, scotch, and tequila, respectively. These different types of spirits smell different, look different, and taste different. However, their alcohol base is identical. If the alcohol were to be distilled, except for certain trace elements, it would be virtually impossible to determine the different sources.

When alcohol enters our digestive tract, it is quickly absorbed. The effect of this is our blood alcohol level rises. One is considered intoxicated when the blood alcohol levels reach a certain point (.08% in the state of California, for example). Metabolized in the liver, the alcohol affects the central nervous system and is a toxic agent. If you drink a lot and drink often, it will affect your health.

Some researchers have suggested that low levels of alcohol, i.e., 1–1½ oz. per day, may, in effect, lower blood pressure and increase the percentage of what are called HDLs (High Density Lipoproteins), which are associated with decreased cardiovascular disease. Whether or not this is actually true, no one really knows. However, since alcohol is the most widely used mood-altering drug available, and since most people like to drink alcohol, my recommendation is that you do so with moderation.

Again, I do not presume that you will be totally controlled all of the time. I therefore encourage you to understand that each time you drink a large amount of alcohol you are challenging your body's capacity to deal with this substance, taking in a lot of calories that you probably don't want or need, and making it more difficult to maintain the weight loss that you have achieved. Make reasonable choices most of the time. If you are going to "over-drink," do so where you are not likely to injure yourself or others by driving, or get arrested or put in jail.

FINALLY

If you find yourself drinking more often than you think is wise, if you find it hard to stop drinking, or if you find yourself drinking to face unpleasant situations that involve people or work, you may have a problem with alcohol. If you do, consider getting professional help.

At this point you're almost home. Food, exercise, and alcohol are being dealt with. Now let's move on to stress and eating.

CHAPTER 7

WHO'S PINCHING YOUR TAIL?
THE STRESS-EATING SYNDROME

"Didn't I ever tell you about my chip drawer?" asked Chuck.

"Chip drawer?" I replied. "No, you didn't. What's a chip drawer?"

Chuck is a sixty-year-old vice president of marketing and sales for an international computer company. We've known one another professionally for a number of years, ever since he first came to see me for some help in getting his weight under control and lowering his cholesterol level.

Chuck's story is a fairly typical one. He had been an athlete in high school and college, playing basketball and baseball. At about 5′9″, he carried 170 pounds quite well. When he was really working out, he had bulked up as high as 180 pounds. Since he has a large frame and is muscular, he was able to handle that weight well. During his thirties he still maintained a reasonable weight. As he got into his forties, his weight began to increase and that increase was fat. There seemed to be two factors involved. First he'd begun to do much more traveling and having many more business lunches and dinners. But what was even more important was that Chuck's work world became a lot more stressful and demanding. There were all these problems to be solved and not enough time to solve them, and Chuck often came home at the end of the day exhausted and with more work to do. What he told me was that as soon as he hit the front door he would begin eating chips, then go to the refrigerator and get some cheese and crackers. It wasn't unusual for him to split a bottle of wine at dinner with his wife. (Guess who drank the most?)

But this was the first time I had heard about his chip drawer. I asked him to elaborate.

"Well, you see, in the kitchen we've got this warming oven."

"Yes," I replied, "but don't you generally use that to keep rolls or bread or plates hot when you're having a dinner party?"

"We used to," said Chuck, "but I decided that it was a great place to keep corn chips. So now we just keep it on warm, I keep it filled, and whenever I get home they're ready to eat."

Chuck is one of the many stress eaters that I've worked with over the years. They tend to be men who are hard-drivers, work long hours, and use food as a way to "come down" without even being aware of it. When I asked Chuck if he really liked chips, he said no. I asked him why he ate them.

"Because," he said, "they kind of take the edge off. As I eat them I can almost feel myself calming down."

"So it's sort of like medicine?"

"What?" he said.

"It sounds to me like the major purpose of your eating chips is to take away the psychological pain you're experiencing—the stress and tension that you have at the end of the day."

"Well, maybe," he said doubtfully.

"Let me ask you another question. The last time you were at a picnic, did they have chips?"

"Yes," he replied.

"Did you eat any of them?"

"Maybe one or two."

"Why only one or two?"

"Because they weren't really interesting to me compared to the rest of the foods."

"How were you feeling at the picnic?"

"I was feeling just great. I was having a marvelous time."

"So," I said, "chips are used primarily when you're feeling bad and are used to make you feel better. Some kinds of food are used like a nonprescription medication simply to make you feel better."

As I reviewed Chuck's food diary (one of the things that I ask my patients to do when I work with them on weight loss), I found out that most of the time when Chuck was really out of control in terms of his eating, the words he used to describe his mood were "strung out," "emotional," "wiped out," "anxious." Chuck actually did reasonably well at meals. It was the unplanned, unanticipated, emotionally based eating that was doing him in, and that's true of many of the men I see.

In order to successfully master the stress-eating syndrome, you need to do the following things:

FIGURE I

1. IDENTIFY THOSE FEELINGS THAT ARE ASSOCIATED WITH UNPLANNED OR UNCONTROLLED EATING.

2. IDENTIFY WHAT IS CAUSING YOU TO FEEL THAT WAY (WHO OR WHAT IS PINCHING YOUR TAIL).

3. IF POSSIBLE, DEAL WITH THE SITUATION THAT'S CAUSING THE DISCOMFORT.

4. IF YOU CAN'T SOLVE THE PROBLEM, USE ANOTHER METHOD TO DEAL WITH YOUR FEELINGS.

5. IF YOU DO EAT, EMPLOY DAMAGE CONTROL PRINCIPLES.

---

1. Learn to identify feelings that are associated with unplanned and uncontrolled eating.

Most of my patients at Scripps Clinic are asked to keep a food diary for at least a week. On it I ask men to keep a record of what they are eating and the reason they're eating. Below you will see three different examples of completed food diaries. Bill, as you can tell, only eats at meals, but the size of his meals is enormous. Emotional issues aren't a major factor in his life in terms of eating, so if you're like Bill, you probably have few problems of this kind.

The second sample is John's, and as you can see, for him stress is a major factor. He not only eats *between* meals when he's upset, but also eats a lot more *at* meals when something is bothering him.

The third sample is Steve's, and Steve is a man with a different problem. As you can see, when he's *stressed* he tends to eat *very little*. But when he's bored, his eating really goes crazy. And so, John and Steve have very different issues they need to deal with in order to master this problem.

Daily Food Record

NAME __BILL__

DATE _____

	TIME WHEN ATE	PLACE WHERE ATE	DOING WHILE EATING	WITH	FEELING WHILE EATING	HUNGER BEFORE EATING	FOOD & AMOUNT
MORNING	8:00	KITCHEN	EATING	FAMILY	GREAT	4	LARGE O.J. SCRAMBLED EGGS (3) 4 TOAST (BUTTER)
							JAM, 4 SLICES BACON HASH BROWNS 1 CUP 2 CUPS COFFEE
AFTERNOON	12:30	REST.	MEETING + EATING	STAFF	GOOD	4	BOSTON CLAM CHOWDER STEAK SANDWICH + FRIES APPLE PIE + ICE CREAM
							1 WINE
EVENING	7:00	REST.	EATING	WIFE + FRIENDS	TIRED	5	BOURBON (2) GOAT CHEESE SALAD VEAL CHOP / PASTA 2 ROLLS
							2 GLASSES WINE CRÈME CARAMEL

HUNGER: In the column labeled "Hunger Before Eating," place your state of hunger as a number from 0 to 5 (0=not hungry, 5=very hungry). If you feel full before eating, write F.

Daily Food Record

NAME __JOHN__

DATE _____

	TIME WHEN ATE	PLACE WHERE ATE	DOING WHILE EATING	WITH	FEELING WHILE EATING	HUNGER BEFORE EATING	FOOD & AMOUNT
M O R N I N G	7:30	REST.	READING PAPER	ALONE	RUSHED	2	O.J. WAFFLE BACON
	9:00	WORK	WORKING ON REPORT	NO ONE	PRESSURED	0	2 DOUGHNUTS
A F T E R N O O N	11:00	WORK	GETTING READY FOR MEETING	O	WORRIED	0	2 CANDY BARS
	12:30	DESK	READING	O	LATE	1	HAMBURGERS FRIES SHAKE
E V E N I N G	7:00	HOME D.R.	EATING	FAMILY	OK	4	SALAD CHICKEN - 2 PIECES FRUITCUP
	11:00	KITCHEN	FINISHING REPORTS	O	TIRED	2	4 SCOOPS ICE CREAM

HUNGER: In the column labeled "Hunger Before Eating," place your state of hunger as a number from 0 to 5 (0=not hungry, 5=very hungry). If you feel full before eating, write F.

Daily Food Record

NAME __STEVE__

DATE _____

	TIME WHEN ATE	PLACE WHERE ATE	DOING WHILE EATING	WITH	FEELING WHILE EATING	HUNGER BEFORE EATING	FOOD & AMOUNT
M O R N I N G	7:30	KITCHEN	EATING	O	STRESSED	4	1 TOAST 1 COFFEE
	10:00	STUDY	WRITING	O	BORED + TIRED	2	2 PIECES COLD PIZZA COKE
A F T E R N O O N	11:30	STUDY	STILL WRITING	1	NOTHING HAPPENING	1	COLD CHOW MEIN PIECE CHICKEN
	7:00	KITCHEN	EATING	FAMILY	WORRIED ABOUT LACK OF PLATES	4	SALAD FEW BITES ROAST MASHED POTATOES
E V E N I N G	11:00	DEN	WATCHING T.V.	WIFE	BORED	1	3 COOKIES SCOOP ICE CREAM CUP GRANOLA

HUNGER: In the column labeled "Hunger Before Eating," place your state of hunger as a number from 0 to 5 (0=not hungry, 5=very hungry). If you feel full before eating, write F.

Now to help you identify what leads to your unplanned or uncontrolled eating, I've included blank copies of a food diary on the following page.

2. Identify what is causing you to feel this way. (Who or what is pinching your tail?)

You may be wondering why I used "Who's Pinching Your Tail?" as the title for this chapter. There is a body of research in the animal psychology literature related to tail pinch. The model is simple. Rats are given full access to food and eat until they're satiated. They are then put into a cage and a small clip-like device is attached to the tip of their tail. That device is connected to a mechanism that can put pressure on the tail while allowing the animal to roam freely around the enclosure. This causes the animals to experience a slight discomfort, which is called the "tail pinch." Researchers have found that this mild discomfort is upsetting to the rats—they are "stressed" by it.

What has been observed is that when this tail pinch takes place, rats begin eating and continue eating in response to the tail pinch. When the pressure stops, the rats stop eating. Sounds familiar, doesn't it? The rat is not hungry, but when stressed, the rat begins eating.

But not all rats. Some rats don't eat under these conditions. As I was watching a film of some research we were doing, I noticed that one rat did something that none of the other rats did. After a few minutes of moving around the cage, this rat looked at his tail and then deliberately tried to remove the tail pinch apparatus. So rather than responding to the stress by eating (as both rats and people do), this rat tried to deal with the source of the stress directly.

So, the thing to do once you've identified the feelings associated with unplanned and/or uncontrolled eating is to ask yourself, Who or what is pinching my tail?

Daily Food Record

NAME _____

DATE _____

	TIME WHEN ATE	PLACE WHERE ATE	DOING WHILE EATING	WITH	FEELING WHILE EATING	HUNGER BEFORE EATING	FOOD & AMOUNT
MORNING							
AFTERNOON							
EVENING							

HUNGER: In the column labeled "Hunger Before Eating," place your state of hunger as a number from 0 to 5 (0=not hungry, 5=very hungry). If you feel full before eating, write F.

Daily Food Record

NAME _____

DATE _____

	TIME WHEN ATE	PLACE WHERE ATE	DOING WHILE EATING	WITH	FEELING WHILE EATING	HUNGER BEFORE EATING	FOOD & AMOUNT
MORNING							
AFTERNOON							
EVENING							

HUNGER: In the column labeled "Hunger Before Eating," place your state of hunger as a number from 0 to 5 (0=not hungry, 5=very hungry). If you feel full before eating, write F.

3. If possible, deal with the situation that is causing the discomfort.

The question to ask yourself is, What can I do to *change how I feel* without eating?

1. If you're bored, rather than eating, deal with your boredom—get involved in a project, read a book, call a friend, or go to a movie.
2. If you're upset because there's a problem bothering you, rather than eating, deal with the problem.
3. If you're feeling down, rather than eating, figure out what you can do to make yourself feel better.

4. If you can't solve the problem, use another method to deal with your feelings.

What can you do besides eating to deal with the feelings and alleviate the need to eat? Well, we've already said that if you're bored, create and/or find something to do that will allow you to feel less bored. If there is a problem that can be solved, solve it. If you're feeling down, try to figure out what you can do to make yourself feel better.

But sometimes it's not that easy and sometimes you continue to feel upset and agitated. So what do you do then? There are two types of activities that are useful in short-term stress management, and these are exercise and relaxation/meditation techniques.

a. Exercise

I've already discussed exercise at some length in terms of its benefits for weight loss and cardiovascular conditioning. I mentioned in that chapter that it also helps with stress. As a matter of fact, one of the things I asked Chuck—the man with the chip drawer—to do, is to go directly to his bedroom when he comes home at the end of the day without going to the kitchen. Chuck has a stationary bicycle in his bedroom and on days that he really feels like hitting his "chip drawer," he will go upstairs, put on a sweat suit, get on his bicycle, and work out for at least twenty minutes. Then he'll hop into the shower and spend another fifteen minutes reading the newspaper before he comes downstairs. Usually by this time his stress level has been lowered sufficiently so that he can just drink a glass of iced tea and wait for dinner.

If you're feeling stressed at mid-day, rather than going to a restaurant and having to choose what you'll order for lunch and facing the temptation of a glass of wine as a "temporary fix," here's what to do. Take a half hour brisk walk to clear your head, pick up a sandwich and a piece of fruit at a take-out deli, and find a comfortable place to eat "alfresco." (This will probably need to be modified if you live in the Northeast and there's a snow storm, during August if you live in Phoenix, and during hurricane season in the South.)

b. Relaxation/Meditation Techniques

One of my patients was attending a convention in Palm Springs that was just not going well and was about to order a major room service meal to make himself feel better (he had convinced himself he was hungry, although lunch had ended only an hour earlier). A colleague stopped by and asked him to join him in the Jacuzzi to discuss a few things. He got out of the Jacuzzi fifteen minutes later and found himself so thoroughly relaxed by the heat and motion of the water, he went back to his room and took a nap for a half hour—something that he had not done in years. But the best part was that he forgot all about eating.

He doesn't have a Jacuzzi at home, so what he does when he's feeling really uptight is to take the hottest shower he can stand for at least ten minutes, change clothes, and sit quietly in the chair for another ten minutes with his eyes closed and soft music playing. He says most of the time this works just fine.

Dr. Herbert Benson, a Harvard cardiologist, has written a book called *The Relaxation Response* (see Figure II) in which he describes a method that he recommends for his patients with mild hypertension. I have suggested it to men whom I see suffer from what I call the "Stress-Eating Syndrome," and my patients have reported it is very helpful.

Finally, for some patients who are chronically stressed and whose stress affects their eating behavior and is causing other health problems, there is a technique called Biofeedback Training.

This is usually done under the direction of a clinical psychologist who specializes in behavioral medicine or medical psychology and usually involves twice-weekly visits to a biofeedback laboratory over a six to twelve week period. For those who might be interested in learning more about these types of techniques, references are provided in Suggested Reading.

5. If you do eat, employ damage-control principles.

You know there are times when nothing seems to work and you're still feeling fairly uptight or upset and need or want something to eat. There is a way to help you manage your eating at least on a short-term basis. What I want to talk about now are two damage-control techniques: the first of these techniques is substitute foods; and the second, portion control.

a. Substitute Foods

Some men find that what they want is simply the release of chewing and swallowing; the type of food isn't that important. If

FIGURE II
BENSON RELAXATION RESPONSE SEQUENCE

1. Sit quietly in a comfortable position.
2. Close your eyes.
3. Deeply relax all your muscles, beginning at your feet and progressing up to your face. Keep them relaxed.
4. Breathe through your nose. Become aware of your breathing. As you breathe out, say the word "ONE," silently to yourself. For example, breathe IN . . . OUT, "ONE"; IN . . . OUT, "ONE"; etc. Breathe easily and naturally.
5. Continue for ten to twenty minutes. You may open your eyes to check the time, but do not use an alarm. When you finish, sit quietly for several minutes, at first with your eyes closed and later with your eyes opened. Do not stand up for a few minutes.
6. Do not worry about whether you are successful in achieving a deep level of relaxation. Maintain a passive attitude and permit relaxation to occur at its own pace. When distracting thoughts occur, try to ignore them by not dwelling upon them and return to repeating "ONE." With practice, the response should come with little effort. Practice the technique once or twice daily, but not within two hours after any meal, since the digestive processes seem to interfere with the elicitation of the Relaxation Response.

you are one of these men, then having a big bowl of air-popped popcorn or one of the light microwave types is a great substitute. It takes a long time to eat, and even a big bowl contains only 200–300 calories (and almost all of it is complex carbohydrates). The other foods that are the classic standbys are chilled celery and carrots. As a matter of fact, Chuck has a big bowl of ice water filled with carrots and celery in his refrigerator. If his exercise hasn't worked well enough or if he's kind of hungry and waiting for dinner, he'll grab a handful of celery and carrots to munch with his iced tea.

Among the other foods that men have reported using that are filling and relatively low-calorie are: hard apples, plain bagels, chewy sourdough rolls, any kind of cold vegetables, or hard cracker breads.

Foods to avoid include nuts, crackers, cheese, potato chips, corn chips, other chips, and, of course, things like cookies, cake, candy, and ice cream.

b. Portion Control

Finally we get to the issue of portion control. And that brings me to the story of Rick. Rick is a forty-five-year-old accountant, married with five children. Rick's wife and his children are biological thins and are not emotional eaters. They are uninterested in food, and if there is a half gallon of premium ice cream in the freezer it will last for weeks.

Not so my friend Rick. Rick comes from an overweight family and has a terrible genetic history with regard to obesity and cardiovascular disease. Rick has been struggling with his weight all of his adult life. He is becoming more successful at meals, but his primary problem is what occurs after dinner as a part of his way to relax or "come down."

Rick will go into the kitchen and serve himself a heaping bowlful of ice cream and then he'll go back and get seconds and sometimes thirds. In a period of thirty minutes, Rick can put away three bowls of ice cream, each bowl containing at least 400 calories, with most of the calories coming from fat and sugar. Rick is about 6'4" and carries 220 pounds comfortably, but his weight is now in the 260-pound range. Still, when you eat 1,200 calories' worth of ice cream a night, it doesn't take a mathematician to say that Rick would have a much easier job of maintaining his weight if he could get his after-dinner stress-eating behavior under control.

So Rick did two things. The first is that now the only frozen dessert in the freezer is nonfat frozen yogurt (a substitute food). Second, I asked Rick to make a major change in *how* he does his after-dinner eating. These are the steps he follows:

1. **Decide what you are going to eat.**
   Rick now puts a single large scoop of yogurt into a **cup** rather than filling a **bowl** to the brim.
2. **Eat slowly rather than quickly.**
   Rick used to inhale his ice cream. Now he's slowed his pace and actually tastes his yogurt.
3. **After you're finished, wait at least fifteen minutes before getting another serving.**
   This gives some time for a physiological response to the food, including an increase in blood sugar level and, according to some recent research, increased levels of a central nervous system endorphin called serotonin. Increased levels of serotonin are related to feelings of satiety.

4. **Then decide if you want more. If yes, go back to Step 1; if no, stop eating.**

    Rick reports he usually has two large scoops of yogurt—only occasionally will he have as many as three. So by the time he's done, he will have had only 300–400 calories without fat rather than 1,200 calories coming *primarily* from fat. In summary, the steps to use for portion control are:

1. Decide what you are going to eat, take a standard serving, and put it on a normal plate or in a cup.
2. Eat slowly, using a fork or spoon.
3. Wait at least fifteen minutes and then decide if you want any more.
4. If no—stop eating and get on with your life. If yes, go back to Step 1.
5. After the third portion, wait at least one hour before deciding if you are going to eat any more.

FINALLY

The next time you open up the package of peanuts on the airplane (because you are bored, not because you like peanuts), or you wind up at 11:00 at night prowling the kitchen looking for cookies, or you come home at the end of the day and begin rummaging around the refrigerator even though you know dinner is going to be ready in fifteen minutes, one question you must ask yourself is: Who or what is pinching my tail and what else can I do besides eat to deal with what is bothering me?

PART II

THE ART

OF

WEIGHT

CONTROL

CHAPTER 8

BEHAVIOR MOD AND ALL THAT STUFF

Stephanie's is a world-renowned restaurant in Melbourne, Australia, located in a lovely large house with a series of small, intimate dining rooms a fifteen-minute taxi ride from the center of the city. I was in Australia for Jenny Craig International, presenting the new video- and audiotapes I developed for their Lifestyle Education classes, and had looked forward to going to Stephanie's since we arrived.

We got there early because I didn't want to be rushed. Stephanie's serves only a fixed price menu, which includes a little something for a starter, then choices of an appetizer, a soup, salad, entrée, and dessert. Because of the size of the meal, I had planned a variation of my "taste everything, eat nothing" strategy and was looking forward to a wonderful evening.

A few minutes after we'd begun eating, a couple was seated behind but slightly to the right of my wife. The woman was slender and attractive. The man could have been attractive but he was a good fifty pounds overweight. As it happened, whenever I looked up to talk to my wife, this couple was directly in my line of vision, and while I'm usually not a person watcher, I simply couldn't avoid seeing how the man was eating.

The house "morsel" arrived and was gone in a flash. Two rolls were buttered and gobbled up. As food was set in front of him, he attacked it furiously. His fork, knife, and spoon were in constant motion. He had ordered conservatively—the asparagus appetizer, the clear soup, salad, the chicken entrée, and the fruit tart for dessert. But it was how he ate that was disquieting. His mouth was always filled with food. Each course was polished off in just a few minutes. When the waitress cleared their plates, hers was always half full, his had not a bit of food left on it. Then he would wait impatiently while his wife continued eating, taking a few more rolls each time.

The waitress could barely keep up with this human eating machine, and even though they arrived some fifteen minutes after us, we were just beginning our entrée when he finished paying the bill. As they walked by us she turned to him and said, "Wasn't that a wonderful meal?"

"No," he replied. "They give you too much food. I can't stay on a diet in a place like this."

As they moved out of earshot, I said to my wife, "He just doesn't get it. He's blaming the restaurant. Obviously, whoever is helping him lose weight has only been teaching him about *what to eat*. They haven't taught him a thing about *how to eat*.

Knowing *what to eat* is not enough. Knowing *how to eat* is equally important. Psychologists use the term *behavior modification* when talking about these things.

In the following pages, I'll be asking you to make seven changes in how you deal with food over a six-week period.

FIGURE I

WEEK 1   A. DUMP THE JUNK.
               B. WEIGH YOURSELF REGULARLY.

WEEK 2   EAT ONLY IN EATING PLACES.

WEEK 3   MAKE EATING A PRIMARY ACTIVITY.

WEEK 4   SLOW DOWN.

WEEK 5   NEVER FINISH ANYTHING.

WEEK 6   STOP EATING WHEN YOU'RE NO
          LONGER HUNGRY.

WEEK 1

a. **Dump the junk. Get rid of the foods that you binge on**
    because they're too tempting or someone or something is
    "pinching your tail."

If you tend to eat peanuts by the handful, ice cream by the carton,
and cheese by the pound, don't have these foods around the house
during your weight-loss phase. If these foods are available, you
will eat them for taste or to relieve tension.

Men are often resistant to this recommendation, believing that
"It's my problem and I should be strong enough to deal with it. I
should just have more self-control." Self-control is not the issue;
environmental control is.

Research indicates that overweight people are much more responsive to food cues and will want to eat when exposed to them.
It's also true that the formula for binge eating is:

$$\text{Binge Feelings} + \text{Binge Food} = \text{Binge Behavior}$$

When men eat out of frustration or for emotional reasons, they
are not likely to gravitate toward broiled fish and green salads.
More often they'll go for cookies, cake, cheese, and the like. If the
food isn't available, you may go out and get it—but it's more likely
that you won't.

One of the things men often ask me is: What about other
members of my family? Why should they have to suffer? Well, if
you are really doing your part, it is not unrealistic to ask them to

be *behaviorally*, not just verbally, supportive. Explain to them that it's much easier for you to stay in control if certain foods are not around. You're not preventing them from eating what they want, just so long as they don't leave the remains for you. By the way, you're probably doing everybody some good by not having high-fat, high-sugar, salty snack foods around. It's to their benefit as well.

But be willing to negotiate. If other family members like oatmeal raisin cookies, but you find them a turnoff, it's okay to have them around, in reasonably small quantities. It's all right to bring home a special dessert when you have guests—just make sure the remainder gets eaten by someone else or brought to the office.

You do have to be credible. If everyone has agreed not to have premium ice cream in the freezer to help you out, and then you bring home a half gallon of Jamocha Almond Fudge and devour it in forty-eight hours, you're not going to get much support. Keeping the house safe will make it much easier for you to stay with your weight-loss program.

b. Weigh yourself regularly. Once a week while you're losing weight, twice a week or more when you're maintaining your weight, but never more than once a day.

1. Losing Weight. The reason you should weigh yourself only once a week while you're trying to lose weight is so that you won't become overly disappointed because you've "starved yourself for a day" and the scale doesn't suddenly respond. Also, it seems much more significant if you've lost two pounds in a week rather than seeing a quarter- or a half-pound weight loss each day.

Do get a scale that's *reliable*. By that I mean it comes up with the same number when you get on it two, three, or four times in a row. It's not as important that the scale be "totally accurate," because wherever you start is where you start. Unreliability means you can't fool the scale by stepping on it in a certain way or finding "the sweet spot." Consumers Union periodically reviews scales. Prices range from moderate to expensive. Since you're not going to buy a scale very often, it's worth your while to invest in a good one. Many men who become serious about weight control will invest in a balance-beam scale like the ones found in a physician's office because they feel more comfortable knowing that what the scale says is what they really weigh.

By the way, there will be times that your weight loss does not appear to match your effort. You must understand that scale weight is a combination of:

1. Fat mass
2. Lean muscle mass
3. Fluid
4. The amount of unprocessed food currently in your system

Each time you weigh yourself you might have lost a bit more weight or a bit less weight than would have been predicted by the number of calories you're taking in and the amount of exercise you're doing. But over a long period of time, it all works out. For an illustration of how this works, see Figure II.

Notice that the weight loss is more rapid at the beginning and slows down as you continue to lose weight. One reason for this is that initial weight loss is a combination of fat, muscle, and fluid, while later weight loss is only fat. A second reason is that as you lose weight you *need fewer calories* and hence the deficit you're creating is somewhat diminished.

2. Maintaining Weight. After you've gotten to where you think you want to be, you must continue to weigh yourself on a regular basis. Some people like to weigh themselves every day, and that's acceptable. What I recommend is that you weigh yourself twice a week, before and after the weekend, so you'll have some notion what your normal variation will be.

The reason I don't suggest you weigh more than once a day,

Figure II

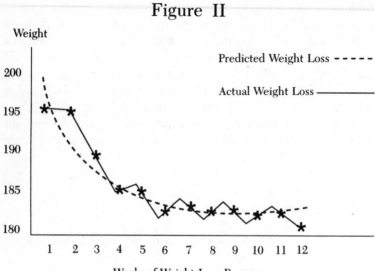

Weeks of Weight-Loss Program

every day, is that you can become scale-neurotic. I know some men who will weigh themselves when they get up, after they've gone to the bathroom, before breakfast, and again after breakfast. Frankly, that gets a little bit weird.

By the way, once you've gotten to a weight that you feel comfortable with, mark that number down. If your weight goes up five pounds for more than one week, immediately go back to weight-loss behavior so it doesn't go out of control.

Everyone wants to know what their ideal body weight should be and there are numerous tables put out by insurance companies that provide ranges for men based upon their age, their height, and their body type. Frankly, these can be rather confusing, since none of them seem to agree. What I'd suggest is that you do one of the following two things:

1. Find yourself an exercise physiologist who will measure

your percentage of body fat either using calipers or an underwater weighing, to help you determine an ideal weight based upon your percentage of body fat. For optimal health, we like to see men below 20% of body fat.

2. If you can't have this done, use the following formula:

106 lbs. for the first 5 ft. and 5–7 lbs. for each additional inch
(morning weight—stripped)
(height without shoes)

For example, a 5'10" man is probably in a good weight range if he weighs between 156 and 176 pounds. If you are at the upper end of this range, then you should have a fairly large bone structure and/or have a fairly high natural level of muscle mass.

These numbers obviously don't apply to those who are professional athletes, because depending on their sport, they might weigh considerably less (if you're a marathoner), or considerably more (if you're a professional football player) and still be healthy.

WEEK 2

Eat only in an eating place.

When I do seminars I ask people what an eating place is and everybody responds in a fairly predictable way—a dining room table, a kitchen table, a kitchen counter, or a restaurant. I then ask a second question: "What are noneating places?" I've gotten a number of creative responses. The favorite noneating place is a car. The second is in bed. Other noneating places include the den, at a desk, the living room, just wandering around the kitchen, the shower, or the garage.

The reason for asking that you eat only in eating places is that it makes eating a *deliberate activity.* It also means that you will be separating a stressful environment (like the desk where you work and feel anxious a good deal of the time) from an eating environment where we'd hope you would be feeling a bit more relaxed. It also decreases the likelihood of random eating, the dazed, wandering munching that often goes on the night that you're trying to finish the big report or are working on your taxes.

By the way, it's perfectly all right to declare some place as a "temporary eating place." For example, one man that I was working with was an architect who would take his lunch but find that most of the sites that he worked were hot and dusty and not at all amenable to a restful lunch. What we did was declare his car an eating place, but only for lunch and only when he was on a construction site. He would then get into his car, put on some music, open up the sun roof, and have a leisurely lunch. However, he agreed not to eat in his car if he stopped at a fast-food restaurant and was zooming from one building site to another.

In a similar fashion, another man decided that he wanted to watch the NCAA basketball finals on the big-screen television in his den. On that evening, he declared the den and a TV table an "eating place," but it was no longer an eating place when the game was over.

WEEK 3

Eat only as a primary activity, not a secondary activity.

The shorthand rule for this is that it's *all right to* **read** *while* **eating** but it's *not all right to* **eat** *while* **reading.** For example, I often leave the house early in the morning and will have breakfast at the hospital or in a coffee shop adjoining my office. I generally have a newspaper with me. If I don't see anybody I know, I'll have breakfast and read the newspaper. In this instance, reading is all right because *eating* is the *primary activity.*

In contrast, if at eleven o'clock at night I'm sitting and reading a novel, is it all right to get something to eat? The answer here would be no because *reading* is the *primary activity*. What I'd be doing is eating something because I'm bored with what I'm reading or tired and really should be going to sleep.

In similar fashion, it's all right to *watch television* while *eating* but not to *eat* while *watching television*. So my friend who declared the den an eating place because he was going to have dinner and watch the NCAA basketball finals was making a positive choice. But if at eleven or eleven-thirty he was simply staring at the news or a late night show, it would not be okay for him to get something to eat then, because watching television is the primary activity.

WEEK 4

Slow down.

Most overweight men don't eat their food, they inhale it. They're usually the first one done and are then surrounded by people eating. If they're at home, they will reach for a second portion, or even a third. In a restaurant, they'll reach for the bread basket. We are not quite sure why overweight people eat so quickly, we just know that they do.

An internationally known weight-loss expert did a research study where he had graduate students go to a number of Chinese and Japanese restaurants and observe whether the non-Asians eating with chopsticks appeared to be normally weighted, underweight, or overweight.

Guess what he found? You're right. *Almost no overweight people were using chopsticks.* The reason was that most non-Asians who use chopsticks are relatively unskilled. Hence, they tend to drop a lot of food, and therefore are forced to eat slowly. Since this doesn't allow them to take it in fast enough, they revert to spoon and fork. (Social science researchers call this a naturalistic experiment.)

In addition to not automatically reaching for seconds or thirds, there's another reason to eat slowly. We're not quite sure what it is that signals the satiety center of the brain that one has had enough food. It's some combination of elevated blood sugar level, a full stomach, brain chemistry, and possibly some psychological sense of satisfaction. We do know that it takes twenty to thirty minutes after a person begins eating for any type of satiety signal to occur.

If you are a rapid eater, you can eat an enormous amount in that twenty to thirty minutes. One man said to me, "By the time my brain says I've had *enough*, I've had *too much*."

There are two ways to slow down, both relatively easy to implement. The first is to change the way you eat at home to be like you eat in a restaurant. That is, have portions and eat in courses, rather than family style where all the foods are on the table at the same time. If you go out for lunch and you have a salad, an entrée, and dessert, what would probably happen is this: the salad would be served first, then your plate would be cleared. A few minutes later would come the entrée, and finally, after the second plate has been cleared, dessert. Eating this way automatically prolongs the amount of time you're going to be eating from five to ten minutes to twenty to thirty minutes, and allows you to leave the table feeling satiated.

Changing the pattern at home will mean being willing to help out, since it's more work to eat this way than to have all the food on the table on platters or in bowls and have everyone help themselves. It also means that anyone who wants more food has to go to the kitchen—good for you, perhaps, but more work for others.

The second way is to eat differently. If you have a slender spouse, friend, or colleague and you eat with them very often, one of the things that you notice is that even though you've started eating at the same time, when you're done, they've barely started. If you watch them closely, you'll notice that they do not tend to eat with a continuous motion. They'll put some food in their mouth, have a sip of water, swallow, then eat some more. What you are probably doing is eating with a continual motion: the spoon or fork is moving non-stop from plate to mouth. A simple technique to change this pattern is:

**Never have a spoon or fork in your hand
so long as there's food in your mouth**

What this translates into behaviorally is taking a spoonful of food, putting it in your mouth, and then putting the spoon down by the side of the plate, chewing, swallowing, then picking up the spoon again. The same thing goes if you're eating something with a fork. Cut off a piece of chicken, pick it up with a fork, put it in your mouth, put the fork down on the side of the plate, and chew and swallow before picking up the fork again.

It may feel awkward at first, but it also felt awkward when you first tried an overlapping grip when swinging a golf club or learned to rotate the tennis racket when hitting a backhand volley. After you did it a number of times, it seemed natural.

The same thing will take place if you eat differently. What you'll find is by eating this way, you'll taste your food more, enjoy it more, and finish when everyone else does.

By the way, my rule for anybody who eats often in Japanese, Chinese, or Thai restaurants is always to use chopsticks. It automatically slows down your rate of eating and the amount of food you're going to eat.

What, you say? You're an expert at using chopsticks? Okay, put them in the other hand!

WEEK 5

Never finish anything.

At some time during your childhood you were told to clean your plate, or take what you want but finish what you take, or don't be wasteful, or other admonitions that encouraged you to be a finisher. Now some people remember these messages more than others, and most overweight people (men and women) fall into this category. So overweight men will finish everything on their plate because they've been taught to. They also tend to finish everything when going to an expensive restaurant. "I paid for it, so I should eat it all." Finally, men will finish things that they like a lot because it tastes so good.

One of the consequences of having the cessation of eating linked to an empty plate is that the person who fills your plate determines how much you're going to eat. That could be the restaurant that serves gargantuan portions, the overzealous host or hostess, even a well-meaning spouse, or you. (Remember, your eyes *are* bigger than your stomach.)

One of the most important things for men who are interested in maintaining their weight is to control portion size. Obviously, you can afford to eat more low-fat foods than high-fat foods. But if you eat enough of anything you can become fat.

If you don't believe it, just consider the fact that *elephants eat nothing but salad—and without any dressing.*

If you are going to learn a new behavior, you've got to stop the old one. Rather than having the empty plate as the cue for stopping, eventually I want you to have a lack of physical hunger as the cue for stopping. But in order to do that, you have to have stopped the behavior of cleaning your plate. So one of the things you need to begin doing is getting into the habit of *always leaving something on your plate.*

It can be a spoonful of cereal, a bit of the dessert, a forkful of salad. If you get into the habit of doing that you will find out that it begins to get automatic and makes it much easier to move on to my last behavioral change rule.

WEEK 6

Stop eating when you're no longer hungry.

First, some quick definitions. Being hungry is not the same as wanting to eat. Remember, being hungry is a *biological* cue characterized by a grumbly stomach, a headachy feeling, or sometimes feeling light-headed. Wanting to eat is a *psychological* cue like a craving, thinking about food, or simply wanting to have a certain taste or sensation.

When I say stop eating when you're no longer hungry, I'm talking about physical hunger, not psychological hunger.

The other thing is that not being hungry is not the same as being full. Not being hungry is the absence of a rumbly stomach, a headachy feeling, or weakness. Being full is kind of like being stuffed. It means that you can't eat any more and it generally means that you're uncomfortable. If you're eating until you're full, you've eaten too much.

FIGURE A

WANTING TO EAT   IS NOT   BEING HUNGRY
THE SAME AS

BEING FULL   IS NOT   NOT BEING
THE SAME AS   HUNGRY

Now remember the last thing I asked you to do is to leave something on your plate. This is simply an extension of that rule. Be aware of how hungry you are when you start eating, and if you're eating right, you're going to be experiencing some of that *physical hunger* before you start eating. If you are aware of when that physical hunger goes away, and you can stop eating then, you've probably had enough.

The secret of being successful here is not to have the food sitting in front of you. If you are in a restaurant, have the serving person clear your plate (and take home that drumstick for a later meal). If you're at home, it means making sure that you take the plate away, because if it stays in front of you, you'll surely finish what's on it.

After a period of time you'll learn how much food you're going to need to feel satisfied. Satisfaction should be the bottom line. You want to stop eating when you're no longer feeling hungry, but well before the time you're feeling full. Satiation and comfort are what you're striving for.

By the way, if you've been overweight for a long time, this may be difficult since many overweight men are almost never hungry because they've been eating so much and so constantly. If you are one of the lucky ones and feelings of hunger return, it makes it a lot easier to monitor your intake based on external rather than internal cues.

FINALLY

From a scientific standpoint, the behavioral control of eating is probably one of the most important strategies in the treatment of obesity and is now seen as an integral part of almost every weight-control program.

The other thing about the behavioral control techniques is that they just make sense.

- If you don't have a lot of stuff around to tempt you, you are less likely to eat.
- Using a scale is like keeping current on your bank balance: it lets you know where you are.
- Restricting your eating to eating places means eliminating casual eating.
- Making eating a primary activity means that it doesn't become a reflex or a habit.
- Eating more slowly allows you to enjoy your food more.
- Never finishing and eventually stopping when you're no longer hungry gives you control of how much you eat.

At this point you probably know more about the science of weight control than 90% of the adult population. In the next section I'll be teaching you the art of weight control, including how to deal with restaurants, or airplanes, or going to a convention, or visiting Europe.

CHAPTER 9

FLYING WEIGHTLESSLY

It used to be that the food served in the back of the plane (read coach or economy) almost always looked bad, tasted bad, and was bad for you. Food served in the front of the plane (read business class or first class) usually looked better, often tasted better, but was not really much better for you. But things are changing. Airlines are beginning to be healthier and are serving things like fish, chicken, whole grain bread, and lighter meals.

The rules for successful flying are:

FIGURE I

1. IF YOU'RE FLYING COACH OR ECONOMY, ALWAYS ORDER A SPECIAL MEAL.

2. IF YOU'RE FLYING BUSINESS CLASS OR FIRST CLASS, EITHER ORDER A SPECIAL MEAL OR CONTROL PORTION SIZE BY TASTING EVERYTHING AND FINISHING NOTHING.

3. PREPLAN SO YOU DON'T EAT AND DRINK BECAUSE YOU'RE BORED.

4. DRINK AS LITTLE ALCOHOL AS YOU CAN.

1. Economy

If you're flying coach, always order a special meal. You can do this on almost every airline so long as you order twenty-four hours in advance. If it's a last-minute flight, you may be able to give as little as six hours' notice.

The usual coach meal is a small salad with regular high-fat dressing, some type of meat with gravy and a wedge of something sweet for dessert. The entire meal is likely to be high in fat, salt, and sugar, not very high in food value, and may or may not taste good. By ordering a special meal you will generally be having something that is prepared by the hundreds rather than the tens of thousands, it's likely to be fresher, and if you order right, not nearly as high in salt, fat, and simple sugars.

Special meals are a limited group of options, which usually include such things as a fruit plate, a seafood plate, a deli plate, a vegetarian plate, a diabetic plate, a low-calorie plate, or a low-cholesterol plate. They are prepared in small numbers and usually show up on the right plane at the right time. As I checked with other airlines, both domestic and international, almost every carrier has some healthy options. At the time of this writing in 1992, American Airlines had developed a series of Heart Healthy Meals. Whatever airline you fly will have a similar program. You may have to urge your travel agent to work a little harder in finding out what your real choices are.

Here are some specific suggestions:

For breakfast, a fruit plate or cold cereal with fruit and low-fat milk (skip the omelette).

For lunch, a seafood plate, a deli sandwich, or a grilled fish entrée.

For dinner, a seafood plate, diabetic plate, low-cholesterol plate, or low-calorie plate.

2. Business or First

If you are flying in the front of the plane you can order a special meal, too, but most people don't because they like to be pampered and eat what they think are more elegant foods. If you fly frequently (weekly or more), go the special meal route. If you fly occasionally, follow these guidelines:

You will usually be served drinks and peanuts and four courses—an appetizer, salad, entrée, and dessert. Start off with mineral water or juice and don't even look at the peanuts. Use the rule of taste everything, finish nothing.

Choose a simple entrée. Often something like steak or roast beef may be your best choice, since everything else is usually heavily sauced or sitting around soaking up its own fat for the last hour. Have some fruit for dessert or just a taste of the hot fudge sundae or the strawberry tart.

3. Preplan

Most people overeat on airplanes because they're bored. Watch the movie even if it's lousy and/or bring lots of things to read. Adventure books, trashy novels, or simple-minded magazines are the best. Relax if you can—work if you must.

If you find yourself with an agreeable companion sitting next to you, talk instead of eating and drinking.

4. Limit Alcohol

The most dangerous part about sitting in the front of the plane is the fact that alcohol is provided free, and it's very easy to take in a thousand calories of booze on a transcontinental flight.

1. Mimosa (orange juice and champagne) upon entry: 150 calories;

2. A glass of champagne before taking off: 150 calories; a glass of white wine with the appetizer: 150 calories;
3. Two glasses of red wine with the entrée: 300 calories;
4. Kahlua coffee with dinner: 150 calories;
5. Cognac after dinner: 150 calories.

Add it all up—that's 1,050 calories.

If you are going to drink at all, stick with the two-drink limit. It is probably best to start with club soda and lime, have one or two glasses of wine with the meal, and/or an after-dinner drink.

FINALLY

It is true that if you are flying during a regular meal hour you may have an actual need for food. The real reason that airlines serve you meals is to keep your mind off the fact that you are sitting in a narrow tube thirty-five thousand feet in the air, are going to be there for a few hours, and are bored out of your skull. It's a distraction.

Most of the food entrées offered in the front of the plane are extraordinarily rich. The reason that the meals are more elaborate (and only slightly more costly) in business class or first class is that since a four-course meal service takes longer to serve than a one-course meal service (read Everything on One Tray at the Same Time)—you feel less bored. More service and larger seats are why you pay a premium.

Since the actual cooking facilities on an airplane are limited, all they can really do is heat up food that has been previously cooked. That's why the best alternative on a plane may well be a steak or roast beef. Although the beef is high in fat, at least there is no high-fat gravy or cheese sauce to deal with.

Overall, you need to think about eating and drinking very defensively on airplanes, simply because your alternatives are not very good. Here are some additional tips that make airline travel more tolerable. (Most of these are already known to the seasoned traveler but may be helpful to the occasional traveler.)

If you can sleep in an airplane, choose a window seat so you have someplace to put your head. If you are restless, choose an aisle seat so you don't have to climb over someone each time you go to the bathroom or feel the need to move around.

Dehydration is a problem in an airplane due to the fact that the air-conditioning system has a tendency to draw moisture. Most health-care professionals recommend that you drink one glass of water for each half hour of flight time. (Now you see why you have to go to the bathroom so often.) By the way, the intake of fluid also fills you up and makes it more difficult for you to stuff away those calories.

If you have not ordered a special meal, particularly if you are in the front of the plane, have a small part of each of the courses but plan not to finish anything. The rule "taste everything, finish nothing" is one widely practiced by experienced travelers. The key to being successful is when you're done tasting, have the flight attendant take the food away. If those egg rolls (read deep-fried salty bread with a few bamboo shoots) and sweet and sour sauce (read 150 calories per tablespoon, mostly fat and sugar) stay in front of you long enough, *you will eat them.* You don't have to eat the meal quickly. What you need to do is get rid of the plate in front of you when you have decided you are done eating, and this means establishing a friendly, cooperative friendship with the person serving you.

Some last words from the science front. Prolonged sitting, particularly for the middle-aged and over, can lead to the development of blood clots in your legs. So physicians now suggest that you walk the aisle every half hour or so.

If you only fly once a year, you don't have to pay attention to any of these recommendations. If you fly more than once a week, you need to follow every one of the suggestions in order to lose weight and maintain it.

CHAPTER 10

RESTAURANT EATING

Steve seemed very interested when I said I was writing a book for overweight men. He told me confidentially that while he only weighed about twenty-five pounds more than he did in high school, his clothes sizes had changed significantly with the extra poundage. His doctor had recently told him that his cholesterol was up in the 280 range and that he needed to both lose weight and change his eating habits if he wanted to avoid getting into serious trouble.

This was a strange time to be talking about weight and cholesterol. We were part of a group of ten people sitting in a beautiful restaurant about to start on a five-course prix fixe dinner, which would probably go on for at least two hours.

Steve is a fifty-year-old married man with three children ranging in age from fifteen to twenty-two. His wife is very health conscious, and dinners at home are generally tasty and prepared in a low-fat way. Unfortunately, Steve only eats at home two or three nights a week. He eats all of his lunches either at his office while *conducting* a meeting, or in a restaurant while *attending* one. Like my friend Fred, whom you met in Chapter 1, he also goes out to dinner for business meetings at least two nights a week, and he and his wife have friends over for dinner at least one night on the weekend.

Steve told me that he had been working hard both to lose some weight and lower his cholesterol. Initially, he tried to "do Pritikin," but after the first couple of weeks he had given up and was back to his old habits. His problem, he confessed, was eating at restaurants.

"How can you expect someone like me to lose weight when I eat out all the time?"

Steve was particularly distressed because he is an attorney who specializes in selling health-care programs to multi-specialty groups of physicians, and as a result of frequent reading knew "everything that I should be doing and how this extra twenty-five pounds is killing me."

Just then the waitress came over to our table and began describing the meal we would be served.

"The first course will be a duck ravioli, followed by a consommé, a Caesar salad, beef Wellington for the main course, and a poached pear with ice cream for dessert."

We had already finished a glass of champagne, so when she smiled enthusiastically and said, "How does that sound?" we all looked a bit stunned by the enormity of the meal being proposed. But we smiled bravely and nodded. As she was about to leave, I caught her eye and said,

"What else could I have for a main course besides the beef Wellington?"

She looked a bit startled and said she'd "check with the chef."

She came back in a few minutes and said there was the option of having broiled salmon or grilled whitefish for the entrée. At that point, a series of questions began to be asked of the waitress by the other nine people (we're all from California and I doubt if anybody in our group had had beef Wellington in years).

What happened was that *nobody* at the table had beef Wellington. There were eight salmons and two whitefish. At that point I raised my hand again and asked about the Caesar salad. Was it made individually or served from a large bowl that had been pre-prepared?

"Oh, no," she said. "We make each salad individually just before it's served."

"Fine," I asked, "could I have very light dressing on mine, no Parmesan cheese, but I would like some extra anchovies."

Once again, requests came from our other nine companions, who ordered changes mainly on the basis of whether people wanted a lot of anchovies or no anchovy. As the waitress was about to leave, I raised my hand once again, and at this point she gave me a somewhat desperate look,

"By the way," I said quietly, "when the dessert comes, how about just the poached pear with no ice cream?" Six other hands went up in the air with nods.

A moment later, Steve leaned across the table and said, "How did you do that?"

"How did I do what?" I replied.

"How did you get her to change everything?"

"Well," I replied, "she didn't change everything. Actually, the only things she really changed were the entrée, and as for the rest of it, I just had her hold back on some stuff."

"But why did you do it?"

"I did it because that's what I generally do when I go to restaurants."

"Make a big fuss and cause problems for everyone?" he said.

"No," I replied. "I just asked them to prepare things and serve them the way I like them."

"What do people generally do?" he asked once again.

"They generally do what I ask them to do. Sometimes it doesn't work out that way, but generally it does."

I went on to explain to Steve my philosophy about eating in restaurants.

"You see, my own belief is that sometimes I can eat healthier in a restaurant than I can at home, or when I'm a guest in someone's home. In a restaurant, I get to order exactly what I want, and have them prepare it exactly how I want it prepared. I only have to deal with the food I've ordered. No one offers me seconds. If there's food left when I'm ready to stop, I can either have it packaged to bring home or have my plate cleared away so I won't be tempted to keep eating.

"So," I concluded, "my theory is that when people are trying to lose weight or are trying to eat healthy, restaurants can be a very safe place if you know how to handle them."

The seven rules for successful restaurant eating are:

FIGURE I

1. CHOOSE A SAFE RESTAURANT.

2. HAVE A PLAN.

3. ORDER EXACTLY WHAT YOU WANT.

4. HAVE THE FOOD PREPARED EXACTLY AS YOU WANT IT PREPARED.

5. NEVER FINISH ANYTHING.

6. WHENEVER POSSIBLE, AVOID BUFFETS. IF YOU CAN'T AVOID THEM, CONTROL THEM.

7. BE SELECTIVE WHEN YOU'RE IN THE FAST-FOOD LANE.

---

1. Choose a Safe Restaurant

One of the things that determines how well you are going to do in a restaurant is the restaurant that you are going to. While you may not always be able to choose the place you eat, understanding what makes a restaurant safe or dangerous will help you in any restaurant situation. Safe restaurants are those that:

- Focus on quality rather than quantity;
- Allow you to order à la carte rather than having multi-course meals;
- Tend to be serene rather than hectic and serve food at a leisurely pace;

- Have a staff and a kitchen responsive to individual requests;
- Tend not to emphasize gravies, cream-based sauces, or use a lot of butter or margarine in food preparation.

Dangerous restaurants are exactly the opposite. Many ethnic restaurants—Italian, Mexican, or even Chinese—are dangerous because they tend to use a lot of fat in food preparation, and many of the entrées are either based on cheese or covered with high-fat sauces.

Restaurants that deep-fry their foods are dangerous as well. And any restaurant that has a salad bar is dangerous because it winds up being a mini-buffet, and there is a tendency to overdo it. It's much better to have a person-sized salad with dressing on the side served at your table than to go through the salad bar and wind up with some lettuce floating on a sea of Green Goddess, covered with bacon bits and Parmesan cheese.

Now I'm not implying, or even suggesting, that you spend your time at dull, boring restaurants. I am suggesting that you be aware of the fact that you are likely to do better if given a choice in a restaurant that serves eight different types of broiled or grilled fish than eight different types of pizza. The more dangerous the restaurant, the more important it is that you have a plan.

2. Have a Plan

There is another essential ingredient in going out to restaurants, and that is planning. The reason that most people have problems is because they don't have any idea of what they are going to order until they get to the restaurant. Then they're put into a situation where they're surrounded by food, social pressure, and a tantalizing menu. At that point, unless you know what to do, you're a goner.

Now, what do I mean by a plan? Let us suppose you're going to an Italian restaurant that you've eaten in before. A plan might go something like this:

I've eaten lightly all day because I knew I was going out to dinner. What I'm going to do is have some club soda and lime to start off with and one or two glasses of wine with dinner. The people that I'm going out to dinner with generally enjoy leisurely dining, so I'm going to have a first course and a salad and an entrée. Since most of the appetizers are pretty heavy, I'll have minestrone soup, get the salad with the dressing on the side, have one roll, and probably order something like a chicken piccata or scampi (which I'll ask them to prepare with minimal butter) or an appetizer-size lasagna for an entrée. Then I'll have a cappuccino and maybe a spoonful of somebody's dessert if it's really good.

If you recall what I've been saying throughout the other chapters in this book, the major thing that you need to do whenever you're eating is to keep the fats down, control alcohol, and have a fair amount of complex carbohydrates.

The other thing is to eat as many courses as other people are eating so that you won't be sitting there without any food in front of you while everybody else seems to be enjoying themselves.

3. Order Exactly What You Want

Ordering exactly what you want means that you first start off by thinking of what you'd *like* to eat and then figure out what *makes sense*. It doesn't do any good to order the lowest-fat, lowest-calorie entrée on the menu and then feel unsatisfied and get mud pie for dessert. The idea is to be *rationally self-indulgent*. So we're going to do two things in this particular section.

First, we'll give you a series of tips that will help you through most restaurant menus. Second, we'll give you some examples of high-fat and low-fat foods that you might find in different types of restaurants.

Remember—the richer the food, the smaller the portion. That is, a half order of lasagna (particularly if what you really want is lasagna) is not likely to be any more harmful than the veal piccata (veal sautéed lightly in a lemon and butter sauce) surrounded by pasta and vegetables. Here are a series of tips that will help you work through the meal.

a. First Courses

Some good first courses include: clams or oysters on the half shell; a shrimp cocktail (watch the cocktail sauce); vegetable appetizers, like asparagus vinaigrette (tell the waiter or waitress to use just a little dressing on it); a steamed artichoke (again, watch the sauce that's served with it), or vegetable-based soups (like minestrone) consommé; bouillon or onion soup without the cheese.

b. Second Course

Salad is a traditional second course, or sometimes even the first course, in most parts of the United States. In Europe the salad is sometimes served after the meal. The problem with the salad is not the salad itself, but the dressing. Salad dressings are used for moisture and flavor. But since most salad dressings are almost all fat, you can take a perfectly good salad that is 50 calories and make it into a 500-calorie monster.

Let me tell you the major secret to eating salads. *Always order the salad dressing on the side.* Then there are three techniques for controlling the amount of dressing you eat.

The first is not to put any dressing directly on the salad. Rather, dip your fork into the dressing, then pick up the salad with the fork that has some dressing on it.

A second approach is to ask the serving person to bring you some wedges of lemon as well as your salad dressing. Take two or three pieces of lemon and squeeze them on the salad (this provides the moisture) and then take one tablespoon of your dressing, pour it over the salad and mix well (this provides the flavor). What you've now done is controlled the amount of dressing that is actually on the salad by wetting the salad with lemon juice. The dressing has been diluted, and some of it will still be in the bowl (do not sop it up with a piece of French bread). You get all of the flavor with few of the calories.

Third, you can simply put on a limited amount of dressing— just enough to give you the taste you want, but not so much as to do you in.

c. Main Courses

The issue here is portion size and fat density. Unless you are a professional athlete in training, you never need more than a regular-size serving. You can probably do with much less, and that's why some people order appetizers for entrées. Another idea is to split the main course with your wife or significant other (but probably not with the new client you're trying to impress).

You probably know by now that the best choices are pasta with a vegetable-based sauce, boiled or steamed lobster or crab, broiled fish, or chicken; next would be broiled, low-fat meat entrées such as London broil, medallions of beef, medallions of lamb, and appetizer-sized entrées like lasagna.

The secret to survival is to not think you have to finish the entire entrée. Satisfy yourself by having some of the accompaniments. Have a whole baked potato (with just enough butter or sour cream for taste and moisture) and half the steak, rather than all of the steak and half of the baked potato. Bring the steak home for another time.

d. Dessert

Think about the last time you went out to dinner. Was it one of the times that everybody ate a bit more than they should? As you finished, did everyone talk about how full they felt? Then what happened? The waiter or waitress rolls over the dessert cart and begins describing each one in loving detail (even though it might have been made in a commercial bakery rather than on site).

Guess what? Half of the people at the table order dessert. Now, you have to ask yourself two questions:

1. Why does the restaurant make such a fuss about desserts?
2. Why do previously full people order them?

It's to the restaurant's advantage to have you order dessert, since they make a lot of money when you do. The reason you've been shown the desserts rather than allowed simply to read the menu listing is that research indicates that the sight and smell of new food tends to stimulate eating behavior even after you're satiated.

So, here's what to do. If there is something you've seen that you simply can't resist, order it, get a few extra spoons or forks, take the first forkful yourself, and pass it around extolling its wonders. By the time it comes back to you, there's usually very little left. It's only the taste that you really want anyway—rarely does the last spoonful taste as good as the first one or two.

The other option is to go for the fresh berries with a bit of liquor. Satisfying, elegant, and completely safe.

Finally, you can just order a nonalcoholic fancy coffee like cappuccino and enjoy.

4. Have the Food Prepared Exactly as You Want It Prepared

Everyone reading this book probably remembers seeing the scene in *Five Easy Pieces* where Jack Nicholson attempts to order an egg sandwich on toast and is told by the waitress that while they do serve eggs with toast, they don't make egg sandwiches. It may also be that every reader has had an experience of trying to have something changed and been told by a waiter or waitress that "there are no substitutes."

Well, times are changing, and restaurants are changing. Most restaurants are becoming very service-oriented. What that means is that a special request is no longer viewed as a burden, and there are fewer times you'll get somebody rolling their eyes or shrugging their shoulders when you ask to have the hollandaise sauce on the side rather than on the asparagus. Not too long ago I was out to dinner with a friend in a rather elegant New York fish restaurant. One of the entrées that caught his eye was the stuffed trout because my friend loves trout.

First he asked the waiter what the trout was stuffed with. He was told it was a combination of chopped shrimp and crab mixed with cheese. He then asked whether or not the trout was pre-prepared or stuffed immediately before cooking. The waiter assured him that the stuffing was put into the trout just before it was prepared. Finally, my friend then asked if he could simply have the trout without the stuffing. The waiter assured him that there should be no difficulty. My friend and the waiter then got into a lively discussion as to whether or not to quickly panfry the trout or put it on the grill. The end result: he got his trout prepared *exactly* as he wanted it.

Having food prepared exactly how you want it also means you can choose the combination of foods and even have some of the food eliminated. Remember my story of the restaurant when I had my Caesar salad with light dressing and no cheese. In a similar fashion, when we go to a Mexican restaurant, my friend Bob will usually order a tostada and asks to have it put on a corn tortilla rather than a flour tortilla, asks them to hold the guacamole, puts on just a few beans (especially if they're refried), a little bit of extra chicken (which he sometimes gets charged for, but sometimes not), extra salad, and then he loads it up with salsa. Bob then gets a custom-made tostada that he enjoys thoroughly and which is just as tasty as the standard kind. He has eliminated about 50% of the fat and calories, which gives him more leeway in ordering the rest of his meal.

My colleague Anthony is always fighting a weight problem and has borderline high cholesterol. When we go out to an Italian restaurant he always wants some pasta, but what he asks for is a half of a side order of pasta with either a marinara sauce (tomato based, little fat) or plain with a bit of olive oil. He then sprinkles on a touch of Parmesan cheese and enjoys the pasta to his heart's content.

Remember, the secret is knowing *what* you want, *how* you want it, and making sure you get it that way.

5. Never Finish Anything

Restaurants serve too much food. If you order a complete meal—appetizer, salad, entrée, and some type of dessert—at a restaurant, you will be given more food than it is reasonable for you to consume at a single sitting. Even if you've made very safe, low-fat choices, the volume of food that even conservative restaurants serve is astonishing. While there has been a recent trend toward "nouvelle cuisine" with an emphasis on quality and presentation rather than quantity, at the time of this writing this trend is beginning to fade and restaurants are moving back toward large portions.

Most of us were told we had to "clean our plates," and as adults we still have a tendency to follow that rule. If you're paying a lot of money for a meal, there is often the need to "get your money's worth." Unfortunately, in attempting to be frugal you sometimes wind up being self-destructive.

So my rule is a simple one. Rather than clean your plate, my suggestion is, *Never, ever finish everything.* A second recommendation is to begin to pay more attention to internal cues (whether or not you're still feeling physically hungry) as opposed to external cues (whether or not the food still looks, smells, or tastes good). As you do this and get more used to not finishing, you'll find that it's easier to do. You'll also find that most of the time you feel better and less uncomfortable as you walk away from the table.

6. Avoid Buffets

In general it is useful to avoid buffets, because these pose major problems to people who are trying to control their food intake. What is a portion when you go to a buffet? Nobody really knows. A portion is as much as you can eat without fully ODing. Sometimes, however, you can't avoid going to a buffet, like at a Sunday brunch. So if you must go, here are some rules to follow:

1. Decide in advance if you are going to go through the buffet line once or twice. Once if they serve only hot food *or* cold food, twice if they serve both.
2. Scan the buffet before you get in line, and as you walk, make a series of specific choices about what you will or will not put on your plate. Focus on what looks particularly good as well as low-fat alternatives.
3. If it's cold food first and hot food second, make sure that the primary cold is salad with a few accompaniments rather than all of the hors d'oeuvres, which tend to be *very high* in fat and calories.
4. When you go down for the hot food, choose either an average portion low-fat entrée (e.g., the chicken), or a small portion of the high-fat entrée (e.g., prime rib). If you're going to have side dishes, have as many as you want, but limit yourself to the equivalent of a tablespoon-size portion per dish.
5. When you return to your table, begin eating slowly and only eat foods that really taste good, leaving on your plate what really doesn't please you.

In the appendix on page 165, you'll find lists of what to order in Mexican, Italian, Jewish, Chinese, Japanese, French, and American restaurants.

7. Be Selective When You're in the Fast-Food Lane

Almost everybody eats at a fast-food restaurant sometimes, because they're convenient, inexpensive, and, of course, fast. But learning how to handle the fast-food scene is critical for survival. First, just because the food is chicken or fish, don't assume it's healthy.

Those chicken nuggets are coated and then deep-fried. Dip them in sauce and you're in high-calorie, high-fat city. A fillet of fish sandwich is also deep-fried and covered with tartar sauce. Definitely not the way to go.

So let me tell you about some ways to survive the fast-food scene. Order a *grilled chicken* sandwich. If you get a hamburger, skip the cheese and bacon. Forget the milk shake. Get an ice tea or a diet soda or some plain sparkling water with lime to drink. If you want french fries, split an order with a friend.

If you order a salad, get low-calorie dressing or watch how much dressing you use. Each of those packets of regular dressing can have as many as 250 calories. Finally, skip the apple turnover and have a piece of fruit or a small nonfat yogurt for dessert as you walk back to your office.

In the appendix that begins on page 187 you'll find some healthy fast-food choices.

FINALLY

One of the best recommendations for people who eat in restaurants frequently, want to be able to have a variety of flavors and textures, and still be in control is to order sauces on the side. In many restaurants, food is prepared in a very simple fashion, either broiled or grilled, and then the sauce is poured over the top. The sauce is often not an essential part of the food preparation. So what you can do is simply ask them to put the sauce on the side of the entrée, or put it in a small dish, which they then bring to the table.

Going out to a restaurant with either friends or colleagues needs to be seen as a *social or interpersonal event with food present, rather than an eating event with people present.* (This is also true for dinner parties.)

Recently many restaurants have become aware of the increased health consciousness of the American public and have begun to cater to it. In some restaurants a menu listing will have an American Heart Association symbol next to it indicating that it's a low-fat/low-sodium choice. Some chains of hotels like the Four Seasons now feature special entrées that are low in fat.

Be on guard, however. There are still some restaurants that list as their "low-calorie special" something as horrendous as a half-pound hamburger, a scoop of cottage cheese, and a cling peach.

Finally, a conversation with a knowledgeable waiter or waitress often pays off dividends. Ask him or her what they would suggest as a very light entrée. Don't say that you are on a diet, just say that you'd like to eat lightly and would like some suggestions from them. Often they will come up with creative alternatives that are not on the menu and can make some recommendations to you.

Restaurants can help you lose weight and keep it off once you know the rules.

CHAPTER 11

CONVENTIONS AND MEETINGS

Jason is a thirty-nine-year-old director of sales and leasing for a medical supply company. During the year he'll attend at least six professional conventions and also have four one-week regional meetings with his own sales staff to acquaint them with new product lines the company is offering and new lease/sales programs that are being introduced.

"It's really rough," said Jason. "There are the awards banquets, speakers' luncheons, cocktail parties up the ying-yang, and just the regular, 'Let's have a drink and talk about it' stuff. I always come back having put on two to three pounds and feeling crummy."

"Well, actually, Jason," I told him, "I've been working on this problem and I think I've got some ideas that you'll find useful. If you want to come back from next week's convention without gaining weight, try doing the following things.

The six recommendations for being successful at conventions and meetings are:

FIGURE I

1. SKIP THE CONTINENTAL BREAKFAST.

2. WHEN ATTENDING A COCKTAIL PARTY:
   A. ALWAYS HAVE A NONALCOHOLIC DRINK IN
      YOUR HAND;

   B. EAT NOTHING;
   C. KEEP YOUR BACK TO THE FOOD
       TABLE;
   D. COME LATE, WORK THE CROWD,
       AND LEAVE EARLY.

3. TRY TO ORDER A SPECIAL MEAL AT THE
    GROUP LUNCHEON OR DINNER. IF YOU
    CAN'T, USE THE TASTE EVERYTHING,
    FINISH NOTHING RULE.

4. WHEN MEETING AT THE BAR:
   A. NO ALCOHOL;
   B. NO NUTS, CHIPS, CHEESE AND
       CRACKERS, OR OTHER ASSORTED
       SNACK FOODS;
   C. WORK AND/OR PLAY.

5. IF YOU COME IN LATE AND YOU ARE
    REALLY FEELING HUNGRY, USE ROOM
    SERVICE TO ORDER A SNACK, NOT A
    MEAL.

6. EXERCISE EVERY DAY AND WEIGH
    YOURSELF EVERY DAY WITHOUT
    FAIL.

1. Why skip the continental breakfast?

Many professional conventions will provide a continental breakfast as a way to encourage people to get up early for the first

meeting and provide opportunities for informal interaction between participants. Unfortunately, in most instances, the continental breakfast consists of juice, muffins, sweet rolls, and coffee. The juice is fine. You know by now that muffins and sweet rolls are fat sponges. You are also likely to be trying to balance a plate in one hand, coffee in the other, trying to talk, and find a place to sit down. These are circumstances that encourage uncontrolled and/or random eating.

A better solution is simply to order a healthy room service breakfast like fruit and cereal and some toast or an English muffin, or go down to the coffee shop and eat there. Finish a few minutes early and you can get to the area where the continental breakfast is being served. Since you've already eaten, just have your last cup of coffee or tea there, wander around, "press the flesh," and use the time for social and business connecting.

2. Cocktail parties

Cocktail parties are a standard part of almost every convention, and they're very dangerous. The environment encourages random drinking and eating in an atmosphere that is difficult to control.

But you can survive a cocktail party easily if you understand that it is really a business event, not a social event.

a. Always have a nonalcoholic drink in your hand.

My recommendation is that you have no alcoholic beverages at a cocktail party because, as you know by now, alcohol clouds judgment and makes it difficult for you to stay in control. However, having a glass of club soda or a soft drink or even some juice in your hand makes you "part of the crowd" and nobody knows whether there's alcohol in the drink or not.

b. Keep your back to the food table.

The next time you're at a cocktail party, observe the people who plant themselves at the food table. They're usually pretty heavy! You'll notice many of the trim people go to the table, take something, and move away, while the others tend to "stuff themselves." Looking at food and smelling food makes it more difficult not to eat it. Keeping your back to the food table makes your decision not to eat a much easier one to follow.

c. Eat nothing.

If you think about what foods are generally served at a cocktail party, they're things like chips and dip, cheese and crackers, cocktail meatballs, hot dogs, rumaki, and peanuts, all high-fat, high-salt foods. It's also difficult to judge how much you've eaten, because the environment makes it difficult to keep count— besides, it's really boring to try to remember how many potato chips you've just had. Plan to eat before you get to the event and/ or plan to have dinner afterward. But don't spend your time eating the cocktail junk food at the party.

d. Arrive late, leave early, work the crowd.

Most professional travelers view cocktail parties as a business event, not a social event, and what they want to do is see and be seen, connect with people, revive old acquaintances, meet new colleagues and/or customers, make arrangements for a future meeting, and move on. The longer you stay at the party, the more likely you are to be tempted to become involved in the booze and food routine. So if the cocktail party is slated from 5:30 to 7:30, get there at 6:15. A lot of people will already be there. Leave by 7:00. You've already spent enough time. If you've eaten before, go out and have fun. If you haven't eaten, go on to dinner.

3. Try to order an alternate meal at group luncheons and dinner. If not, use the taste everything, finish nothing rule.

A few years ago I was a speaker at a luncheon. Usually, I don't eat very much if the meal precedes the talk, since I find that I do better talking with people around me and preparing for my talk rather than trying to deal with a lot of food. This time I was talking before the meal.

After my hour talk I was really hungry, but when lunch arrived it was crepes filled with cheese and seafood, covered with a heavy cream sauce. I was sitting at the head table facing five hundred people, so I simply smiled and began moving the food around on my plate.

As I looked to my left, I noticed that someone was being served a fresh fruit plate. After the luncheon was over, we were chatting and I asked him how he had managed to get a different meal.

He told me that he had been advised to go on a low-fat diet by his physician. While he was able to manage in most situations, he found that the preset meals at banquets, where the restaurants were trying to serve hundreds of people at the same time, were foods prepared in advance and then kept warm until serving. These meals resemble standard airline entrées—high in fat and sodium.

"So what did you do?" I asked.

"Well, I'd just call up a day or two before, talk to the maître d' or the catering manager, tell them I'm attending the luncheon but had some dietary restrictions and needed to know what was being served. If it was something like broiled fish or a salad, I'd just ask for some sauce or dressing on the side. If it was something awful, I'd ask for broiled chicken, or a fruit plate, or a vegetable plate. In almost all instances, people are very helpful."

"Does anybody give you a hassle?"

"Rarely. If it becomes too much trouble, I simply say forget it and not eat very much at that meal."

If you can't order a special meal, don't sweat it. If the food is reasonable, eat it. If the food is awful, eat the salad, some bread, pick at the entrée, and spend your time talking and doing business. Grab a turkey sandwich later.

4. Meeting at the bar

One of the standard lines at every professional meeting is, "Let's get a drink after the session and we'll have a chance to talk." Going to the bar to get a drink is a natural part of attending a convention. Here's what to do.

a. No alcohol

We've already talked about the two-drink maximum. My recommendation is take your alcohol at meals rather than at the bar. So sit down, order a club soda or a diet drink, or if you're really feeling hungry, some juice. Juice will cut your hunger for an hour or so to allow you to wait comfortably until the next meal.

b. No nuts, chips, cheese and crackers, or other assorted snack foods

The second thing you should do is avoid those snack foods that are put on the table. Generally, they're peanuts or cheese and crackers, or chips, etc. All are very high in fat and very high in salt. Because of their high salt level, they encourage people to drink more.

Just remember, a small handful of peanuts could be a few hundred calories, 70% of those calories coming from fat. A few crackers and cheese can easily add up to 400–500 calories, with most of the calories coming from fat. Since there are so many other opportunities for you to be confronted with food, my suggestion is that you scrupulously avoid the bar snack and eat only at meals.

Here's what can happen if you don't watch it. A patient came back from a five-day professional meeting in Hawaii having gained six pounds and was absolutely astounded. He swam every day, ate carefully, but as we continued to talk, he mentioned that he had stayed at the Mauna Kea Hotel on the big island of Hawaii. The bar has an evening ritual, which included a group of native Hawaiian musicians playing authentic music as the sun sets.

Phil and his colleagues would go there every evening and sit and listen to the music. Sometimes he'd get a drink and sometimes he didn't. The bar puts bowls of macadamia nuts on each table and also brings a tiny hibachi and hors d'oeuvres on skewers, which can be cooked over the flame. What Phil didn't know is that macadamia nuts are very calorie dense, approximately 250 calories per ounce.

He also didn't pay attention to the fact that the hor d'oeuvres were cocktail franks and ham separated by green olives, which are also very fat and calorie dense. Phil would often have a couple of bowls of peanuts and two or three orders of hors d'oeuvres. Given the fact that he was already eating more than normal at regular meals and adding a couple of thousand extra calories a night in peanuts and hors d'oeuvres, it was pretty easy to put on six pounds over a five-day period.

c. Work and/or play

Not being distracted by whether you're eating too much or by the effects of alcohol, you'll probably find it's easier to focus on what's going on. You'll be sharper if you're having a business discussion and less distracted if it's primarily social.

By the way, don't spend any time talking about why you're not drinking alcohol or munching on the snack foods. If anyone asks, just say something like, "I don't want to ruin my appetite for dinner," or "I don't really feel like a drink right now."

5. If you arrive late and you are really hungry, use room service to order a snack, not a meal.

Lots of times when you're attending a convention, the schedule gets fouled up. You arrive at your hotel at 10:00 P.M. and you had lunch at 1:30 that afternoon. Or, you're socializing with people and don't have dinner, or there is an evening session that doesn't end until 9:00 P.M. There could be many reasons, but the result is you wind up in your room somewhere between 9:00 and 11:00 P.M., having eaten nothing since lunch and feeling truly hungry.

What to do? My suggestion is that you **don't order a meal.** You just want to have enough food to allow you to come down from the stresses of the day, and to have enough calories in your system to allow you to fall asleep without being hungry. So you have a number of choices: a bowl of fruit, and an English muffin and some herb tea; a chicken sandwich and some mineral water; or if you're really feeling self-indulgent, even a small, simple dessert like a scoop of ice cream or a strawberry tart and some decaf coffee.

Now while I generally recommend that you skip dessert, sometimes you just *feel* like having something sweet—and in this case you're having the dessert *as* the meal rather than *with* the meal. The dessert is not likely to be more than a few hundred calories and will do the trick. It will make you feel good, get rid of the hunger, and allow you to fall asleep without having a full meal to digest.

6. Exercise daily and weigh yourself daily.

Remember, being at a convention is very demanding. You're working hard, your time is not controlled, your eating is not controlled, and there are numerous temptations. Exercise and daily weighing are mandatory.

a. Exercise.

Remember, exercise not only burns excess calories but lowers stress. One of the best times to exercise is to use one of the non-preplanned meal times. That is, if the morning is packed and there's a break from 12:00–1:30, and no luncheon planned, then use the time to either go to the gym in your hotel or go take a forty-five-minute walk, come back, change clothes, grab a couple of pieces of fruit, and relax until the afternoon sessions start.

b. Weigh daily.

Being at a convention is a time to maintain your weight, not to try to lose, but you can't do that unless you know how things are going. Be certain you weigh yourself every single day, either by using the scale in the gym or finding a pay scale somewhere close. Just make sure you monitor your weight so that you don't have the experience of my friend Phil and come home six pounds heavier.

FINALLY

Conventions and meetings are very hard work. It's important not to view it as a vacation, even though there may be some social aspects. The goal is to be effective, enjoy yourself, and not gain weight.

If you only go to one or two meetings a year, you can relax a bit, although I think that the guidelines make very good sense. If you attend meetings or conventions more than a half dozen times a year, it's mandatory that you pay attention to the guidelines.

CHAPTER 12

How to Avoid Gaining Ten Pounds on a Seven-Day Trip

I'd been working with Dick, a forty-two-year-old attorney, for almost a year. In that period of time he had lost approximately forty pounds, achieved his lifelong goal of being trim, and was feeling better than he'd felt since he was seventeen. I'd not seen Dick for more than a month, but when he did stop in my office for a touch-base meeting, he'd regained almost ten of the pounds he had previously lost.

When we began discussing what had occurred, he reminded me that the last time we had met he'd told me that he was going to Chicago for a couple of weeks to do a little bit of business and have a lot of fun, and that he would be back to see me when he returned.

"What happened?" I asked.

"Well, I guess I just blew it. The hotel said they had an exercise room. But when I got there it was being refurbished and wasn't available. That was the first thing. Then I somehow got into a different mentality. Like, I was on vacation, so I should be able to eat whatever I wanted. Then, I stopped weighing myself. When I got home I found that I had put on almost five pounds and I was so 'P.O.'d' that I just said the hell with it. If we hadn't had this appointment scheduled, I might've just thrown in the towel."

"Okay, Dick," I said. "Part of what went on is my fault, because

126

we really didn't spend the time talking about your trip and helping you to plan so that you'd have a more successful experience."

I then proceeded to tell Dick my three rules for successful travel.

FIGURE I

1. SET ACHIEVABLE GOALS WITH REGARD TO WEIGHT, FOOD, AND EXERCISE.

2. IF YOU'RE GOING TO BE GONE FOR MORE THAN THREE DAYS, WEIGH YOURSELF ON A REGULAR BASIS.

3. CHOOSE THOSE HOTELS, CRUISE SHIPS, AND AIRLINES THAT WILL MAKE WEIGHT CONTROL A PLEASURE.

---

1. Set achievable goals with regard to weight, food, and exercise.

a. Weight

It doesn't make a lot of sense to plan to lose weight while traveling. Your schedule will be disrupted, you'll be eating in new and unfamiliar surroundings, and whether you're away on business or pleasure, your time is likely to be precommitted to a number of activities. Given these circumstances, trying to continue to lose weight is not realistic.

On the other hand, and this is *critically important*, being away from home does not give you license to revert to your previous eating and exercise behavior, because if you do, you're likely to not only regain much of the weight that you have fought to lose but you will also begin to reintroduce behavioral patterns that you have fought hard to change.

The goal is to return home weighing no more than you did when you left. How you deal with food and exercise will determine how successful you are in achieving this goal.

b. Food

It's important to be able to sample the regional food in the area that you're visiting, because part of the fun of traveling is to be able to have new eating experiences. If you are in Italy, you are going to want to try the pastas. If you are in France, you'll want to sample some of the wonderful breads, rolls, and cheeses. If you're in New Orleans, you're certainly going to want to taste the Creole cooking. And if you're in New York, you're going to want to have at least one visit to a traditional deli for a corned beef sandwich with creamy coleslaw on the side.

Now you might be thinking that this sounds contradictory, because many of the foods I've mentioned have previously been identified as being high in fat. Well, yes and no.

First, by not trying to lose weight, you've given yourself a few more options in terms of how much you can eat, because you're no longer trying to create a calorie deficit. As a rule of thumb, if you multiply your current weight by twelve, that will give you the approximate number of calories that you can eat while maintaining your weight. Second, I'm not suggesting that you overindulge at every meal, only that you give yourself the opportunity to become part of the culture in terms of food.

In general, travelers should plan one main meal and two micro-meals a day. The main meal is usually dinner, but it might be lunch. The micro-meals should be smaller servings of simple foods that will sustain you.

For example, a few years ago I went to Paris with my family and we stayed at a hotel that offered breakfast with the room. Breakfast consisted of a basket full of croissants, brioches, breads, wonderful jams, sweet butter, cold cereal, and café au lait. The first day I ate one of each—a brioche, a croissant, some bread, and cereal. From then on I changed my routine so that mornings generally involved eating cold cereal, either half a brioche or half a croissant, a piece of bread (no butter), jam, and two cups of that wonderful café au lait. Lunch often consisted of picking up three or four pieces of fruit at a local outdoor stand, a large bottle of sparkling water, a loaf of crusty French bread, and just a few slices of cheese, which we'd share amongst the four of us. In most instances, dinner was the main meal of the day and here we would indulge a bit more.

The rule was to allow only one of the four courses to be rich. If I was going to have a bowl of onion soup loaded with cheese, the salad was ordered with a simple oil and vinegar dressing, the entrée would be something like a coq au vin (chicken cooked in wine) with steamed vegetables on the side, and dessert was always one absolutely gorgeous pastry, but with four spoons. The two-drink per day maximum was almost always followed. In France it was wine, as it might be in California, while beer might be the better choice in the Netherlands or Denmark.

If we were going out to a concert or the theater in the evening, we would generally have our main meal at lunch and then have some bread and salad and some type of sliced meat from a charcuterie (basically a take-out deli), and then go for coffee and a sweet after the theater. Notice that I did not mention a sliced turkey sandwich with mustard, only because that would be an uninspiring choice of food while in the gourmet capital of the world.

So the general rule is, go with the region, have one main meal, have two micro-meals, and indulge but in a responsible fashion.

c. Exercise

I go skiing perhaps twice a year. To be more truthful, I go "falling" twice a year, because that's where I spend at least half the time when I ski. For anyone who skis, and particularly for anyone who skis badly, you know how much effort it takes simply to put on the boots and skis, get to the chair lift, wait in line, get on and off the chair lift, take a run, and then go through the routine again.

When I go skiing, I sometimes do additional exercise and I sometimes don't. If I'm at a hotel that has an exercise room, I may spend a half hour on the stationary bicycle at the end of the day just to get the kinks out and because it's a way to unwind. I probably won't do it every day, because my legs are already taking a beating on the slopes. If there is a heated pool, I might swim a few laps, but I'm not going to be fanatic about it. The reason is that I know that I'm using a lot of calories skiing and I'm not that concerned that I'll lose any aerobic fitness if I don't do my regular exercise routine for a week or ten days.

However, the situation is quite different when I go to New York. Generally, I'm there for a series of business meetings or to attend a professional convention, or perhaps I'm there on holiday. There are going to be many opportunities for eating and there's nothing that's purely physical built into my day.

In New York, I do two things. First, I try to stay at a hotel that has a well-equipped exercise room and I exercise every single morning that I'm there. If the weather is lousy, I'll use a stationary bicycle. If the weather is good and I'm in a hotel near Central Park, I'll usually "run the reservoir," because it's fun, it gives me an opportunity to experience a different part of the New York culture, and I sometimes run into old friends.

Finally, weather and scheduling permitting, I will walk to almost all of my meetings, even if it takes thirty minutes or more to get there. It gives me a wonderful way to see the city and it adds to my calories out, therefore giving me more latitude to experience all the wonderful New York restaurants. On the way to a meeting, I might get a soft pretzel from one of the street vendors and have it for lunch.

So the general rule for exercising is that if the trip has a lot of built-in physical activities (e.g., skiing, hiking, a tennis camp, scuba diving), then whatever additional exercises you do are optional. If the trip is basically sedentary with lots of eating opportunities (i.e., a cruise, visiting a city like Chicago, London, or Tokyo, or taking a driving vacation with lots of sitting), then exercise should be mandatory and is best done first thing in the morning. A second, briefer exercise period at the end of the day is not a bad idea, either.

2. Weight yourself on a regular basis.

There is nothing more upsetting than coming back from an extended vacation and finding that you've gained five or ten pounds. One of the ways to avoid this is to use the scale even when traveling, and I'll introduce you to three different ways that you can do this. The major goal in all of these is to make sure that you don't gain any weight unknowingly while you are away.

a. If you are only going to one place

The first morning of the first day that you are in a new city, find a scale and weigh yourself on it. It doesn't make any difference where the scale is: in the gym at your hotel, or in Europe, there are always scales at the train station, or simply a pay scale a block from the flat in London that you've rented for the week.

Don't worry about what the scale reads, because it will probably not match your scale at home. For example, if it says that you weigh 175 pounds, write that number down. Then every day that you're there, weigh yourself on the same scale. If the number goes up, it means that you're gaining weight and you better alter either your eating or your exercise. If it goes down, you can either continue doing what you're doing or give yourself a bit more latitude in terms of food choices. If it stays where it is, then you're doing everything right.

b. Traveling from city to city

When people take extended vacations, they'll often wind up being in three or four different places. The rule here is the same but somewhat modified. The first day that you arrive in a city, find a scale and weigh yourself on it. Try to weigh yourself every day that you are in that city. Be *certain* that you weigh yourself the day that you leave. So long as you weigh the same the first day and the last day, you're doing fine. If the scale has gone up two to three pounds, it means that you've gained two to three pounds.

You are now on notice as to what to do when you arrive in the next city. Find a scale there and weigh yourself, and follow the same routine. So long as you weigh the same amount on the same scale when you leave a city as you did when you arrive, you are doing just fine. If you wind up gaining weight each time you leave, and you are going to be gone for a long period of time, you're getting into trouble. Thus you'd better begin modifying your eating and/or exercise behavior as a result of the immediate feedback that you are getting, and stop gaining weight.

c. For people who take driving vacations or go to a camp site for a week or more

Obviously, if you are hiking through the mountains you're not going to have an opportunity to weigh yourself. But if you're driving from place to place and/or are staying outdoors in one location, like a camp ground, I suggest that you purchase a travel scale. These can be ordered from places like Hammaker-Schlemmer, the Sharper Image, or Sears; they are small and light, and while they're not as accurate as the scale you use at home, they are adequate for the task.

Weigh yourself every morning to make certain that you are not doing anything that's too self-destructive. I know this may sound like more trouble than you think it's worth, but believe me: when you come home after a week or more, get back on your home scale, and verify that you've either maintained your weight or lost a pound or two, you'll thank yourself for having made that decision.

3. Choose those hotels, cruise ships, and airlines that will make weight control a pleasure.

There is a lot of competition for your business these days, and one of the ways that the travel industry competes is by offering health and fitness options. Given the choice between an airline that allows you to preorder special low-fat meals and one that doesn't, select the airline that gives you a choice.

When considering what hotel to stay in, inquire about their exercise facility. Don't depend on what it says in the guide book. Call the hotel directly and ask them specifically about their exercise facility: how large it is, what hours it's open, what equipment it has, and, if possible, talk to the person who manages it to find out what other perks (like classes or a fitness instructor) are available and at what cost. Many times the description in the brochure or the tour book will be overly generous. I suggest that you check it out before you make your reservation.

Cruise ships have become a favorite vacation choice for many people. You only have to unpack once, everything is prepaid, and the ports of call can be very interesting. You usually have your choice of cruise lines—many service the same parts of the world. In making your choice and comparing amenities, consider the extensiveness of the exercise facility and programs, and the willingness of the kitchen to prepare meals that are high in quality, appearance, taste, and low in fat.

Some ships specifically emphasize this feature. For example, the *QE 2* exercise facility is run by the staff of the Golden Door (a very special health resort in California). Their menu also features spa cuisine-type meals, which are specifically designed to be low in fat, sodium, and calories. At this time, most cruise lines say they have health and fitness plans. As you investigate, you'll find that some are much more committed to the ideas of healthy living, exercise, and food than others. Make the choice that supports your goals.

FINALLY

A number of men and women that I've worked with over the years wind up losing weight while they travel and do so with little effort. The reason is that these people are usually "stress eaters," and when away from home and many of their work and personal burdens, find themselves naturally reverting to a more healthy and more relaxed way of eating and exercising.

One man who came to talk with me before he left for a three-week trip to northern Italy was concerned that he would not be able to handle the wonderful food that he would be exposed to. I gave him a few suggestions and sent him on his way.

He came back to see me a few days after his return and told me that while he was on the trip he had actually lost a total of seven pounds over three weeks, and he did this with very little effort. He found himself eating only at meals, not snacking out of boredom, and in addition to taking a morning run six days a week, as a tourist, he walked through most of the cities that he visited.

When he got on the scale, however, I noted that his weight was only two pounds lower than it was before he had left. I asked him what happened to the other five pounds. He reported that since he had been home he had reverted to his old pattern of stress eating, and since he had a lot of work to do was "eating everything in sight." We reestablished a number of behavioral controls and he was able to get back on his program.

Sometimes it's easier to be away than it is to stay home.

CHAPTER 13

FOR THE WOMEN WHO LOVE THEM

As I have become known for treating overweight men, many women have called me. They usually begin by asking a variation of the question: "Dr. Shaevitz, what can I do to *get* my husband/ boyfriend/father/son/colleague (choose one) to lose weight?"

The following are some typical inquiries.

From a woman patient:

Dr. Shaevitz, I'm really worried about my husband. He's got high blood pressure, he's had two episodes where blood vessels in his eye have burst, he has high cholesterol, and he's sixty pounds overweight. I know he has to lose weight and so does he, but every time I bring up the subject he says, "I'll take care of it when I'm ready to, and I'm just not ready yet."

From a 26 year old single woman:

I'm really worried about my dad. He's gained about fifty pounds in the last few years and he's beginning to pay the price. While he still plays tennis two or three times a week, he just looks tired. When I come over for dinner, he eats non-stop. The one night I was there he had two drinks before dinner and finished almost a whole bottle of wine by the time the meal was over—all by himself. Mom tells me that it's even worse when they go out. What can I do to get my dad to come in and see you?

From a woman friend:

My brother is almost eighty pounds overweight, and his wife says he does things like go out to the garage where he keeps ice cream and eats it out of the carton. It's particularly bad when he's worried or working on a project. We talk about it constantly and he always agrees that he should do something about it, but so far he hasn't. I'm at the end of my rope. What can I do to help?

From a mother:

Dr. Shaevitz, I don't know if you remember me but I was in one of your programs almost five years ago. I lost thirty pounds and I've kept the weight off. But I'm really worried about my son and he's only thirty, but he's at least fifty pounds overweight. He does things like go on a crash exercise program and one of those liquid fasting programs. That generally lasts for a few months. He loses twenty-five or thirty pounds and then almost always injures himself, or gets bored, and then stops. I know that he's lost and gained at least 100 pounds in the last few years. What can I do?

If you are reading this chapter, you are probably concerned about an overweight man in your life. This chapter was originally written primarily for wives and significant others. However, in conversations with other women—mothers, daughters, sisters, friends, and even colleagues—I've found that they, too, want to help men they care about get healthier, live longer, and lose weight. So the information in this chapter is relevant for these women, too.

To begin with, getting healthier and losing weight are his, not your, responsibility. Neither you, nor I, nor his physician can *make* him do anything. It's all up to him. Sometimes women try to change the men in their lives because they feel responsible for them. But people, and especially men, don't change for others. They change when they are ready or when they are inspired.

The focus of this chapter is on what YOU, a woman, *CAN DO AND SAY* that will be effective in supporting a man's staying on the Lean & Mean Regime, including:

1. What attitudes, comments, and behaviors *are not* productive and *why*
2. What attitudes, comments, and behaviors *are* productive and *why*

I'm assuming that you have not read any of the other chapters in this book, so let me first give you some basic information about male obesity and health. Obesity is an independent factor for the development of a variety of medical problems, including cardiovascular disease, diabetes, gallbladder disease, musculoskeletal problems (bad knees, ankles, or backs), and sleep apnea (a disorder characterized by loud snoring and frequent episodes of gasping for air).

When most men get fat, they store their fat around their midsection (the characteristic apple shaped or "beer belly"). What's important to know is that this abdominal fat storage is linked to increased frequency of heart attacks. So the man who carries twenty or thirty extra pounds (or fifty or a hundred extra pounds) around his middle is more likely to have a heart attack before the age of sixty than you are. *Fat men die young.*

The *good news* is that losing weight, even a moderate amount, will significantly decrease the severity of any of these medical problems and increase a man's life span. But he has to keep the weight off—losing and gaining weight may be worse than staying fat. That's why Lean & Mean is a life-long, not a short-term, program. But it's also a simple program, because I've only asked men to make four changes.

First, I've asked men to eat differently. The single dietary change I ask men to make is to *decrease* the amounts of *fat* and *increase* the amounts of *complex carbohydrates* they eat. That means eating *less* red meat, cheese, butter, creamy salad dressings, rich desserts, and the like, and eating *more* vegetables, fruits, breads, pastas, and cereals.

Second, I deal with exercise. It has been found that a man's level of physical activity is associated with his health status. So the Lean & Mean Program encourages his gradual involvement in an exercise program. Going to a gym once a week or playing golf on the weekends are **not enough.** Exercising forty-five minutes to an hour a day, five or six days a week during weight loss, and thirty to forty-five minutes a day, four to five days a week for weight maintenance is what I've recommended.

Third, I've asked men to drink less alcohol. Alcohol consumption is associated with major medical problems, including cardiovascular disease and various types of oral cancer. It is also a patent source of calories, makes it more difficult for men to control their eating, and inhibits fat metabolism.

Fourth, I've focused on why and where men overeat and provided them with some coping skills for dealing with problem eating situations, including when they're feeling stressed; eating at restaurants, cocktail parties, and business lunches; and how to eat healthily while on vacation, when flying, and even at conventions.

The Lean & Mean Routine can be summarized by the acronym **SAFE**—

- Reduce   **S**tress eating
- Control   **A**lcohol
- Decrease **F**ats
- Increase **E**xercise

THE BRUTAL FACTS ABOUT MEN AND THEIR WEIGHT PROBLEMS

- **Most men hate being fat.** They know they look bad, feel worse, are less sexual, and are likely to get sick more frequently and die prematurely of a heart attack or stroke.
- **Most men hate diet books, diet food, diet programs, and dieting.** They know little about calories, nutrition, or healthy eating. Even though more men than women are overweight, women outnumber men in their dieting behavior by a ratio of 4 to 1.
- **Most men hate admitting they have "a problem" of any kind.** Men are less willing than women to seek assistance from others, including health and mental health professionals. It's not manly to get help; it's embarrassing and humiliating.
- **Most men hate being told what to do.** Men are always looking out for signs that someone is trying to tell them what to do and how to do it. This goes totally against their grain because being competent, self-sufficient, independent, and knowledgeable are at the heart of a man's having self-respect and feeling manly.

SOME OTHER THINGS YOU MIGHT WANT TO KNOW

I've been professionally involved in helping people lose weight for almost twenty years and I currently direct the Eating Disorders Programs at Scripps Clinic and Research Foundation. Men are referred to me by their physicians because they have major medical problems, such as cardiovascular disease, diabetes, or sleep apnea, and need to lose weight for these reasons. Some men seek me out on their own because of my specialty in treating male obesity. According to national surveys, more men than women are overweight. Yet 80% of the people who join weight-loss programs or come to weight-loss clinics are women. How come?

First, there are cultural differences. If a man is twenty-five pounds overweight, who cares. If a woman is twenty-five pounds overweight, everyone cares! Research shows that women are more likely than men to be depressed, denied promotions, and even admission to selective colleges if they are moderately overweight. Women are, therefore, much more motivated to be slender than are men. Women are also more health conscious and prevention oriented than men.

But the real reason why most men don't go to weight-loss programs is that men hate to ask for help. Most men like to feel they can do everything themselves, and asking for help for anything is unmasculine. That's why men are attracted to programs that offer instant cures—fasting programs, "magic" milk shakes, or diet fads such as eating hard boiled eggs and grapefruit.

Even though we've become a dual-career society, most men still don't do much cooking and don't know very much about nutrition. They tend to eat out a lot. If they live alone they eat whatever's easiest to get or cook. One single man told me that if it were not for pizza, take-out Chinese food, and microwave ovens, he might just starve. If a man lives with a woman, he eats what she puts in front of him or what they cook together.

Daniel Evan Weiss, in his book *The Great Divide: How Females and Males Really Differ*, reports that 90% of married women say they do most of the cooking as opposed to 15% of married men. Only 7% of women almost never cook, while 35% of men almost never cook. Finally, 77% of working mothers say they prepare dinner alone while only 16% say their husband prepares it alone.

I'll be making a number of suggestions regarding food preparation. So, if the relationship with the man in your life involves more sharing of meal preparation or if *he* does *most* of the cooking, then some of my recommendations might not be as relevant for you. But if you prepare meals, then cooking healthy food in reasonable quantities without making it seem (as one man put it) "artsy fartsy" is a good idea. I suggest that portions be substantial: a **large** salad, a **large** baked potato, a **large** vegetable dish, a **generous** serving of fruit with some sorbet for dessert. Food can be prepared in a de-fatted way—yogurt on the baked potato rather than butter; chicken or fish rather than steak. In a sense, doing many of the things you already know about.

Specific recommendations will be found below. In order to follow the format that I've used in the rest of this book, each of these recommendations is followed by a discussion.

FIGURE I

1. DON'T TELL ANYONE, AND I MEAN ANYONE, INCLUDING YOUR MOTHER, SISTER, BEST FRIEND, BOSS, OR COLLEAGUES, THAT HE'S TRYING TO LOSE WEIGHT.

2. DO TALK WITH HIM IN A WAY THAT MAKES HIM WANT TO LISTEN.

3. DO HAVE LOTS OF SAFE FOOD AROUND.

4. DON'T BUY "DANGEROUS," HIGH-FAT SNACK OR OTHER FOODS HE TENDS TO EAT WHEN HE COMES HOME FRUSTRATED AT THE END OF THE DAY, OR WHILE WATCHING TELEVISION IN THE EVENING, OR WHEN HE'S WORKING ON A PROJECT LATE INTO THE NIGHT.

---

5. DON'T SERVE HIM ANYTHING THAT LOOKS LIKE "DIET FOOD," OR TINY PORTIONS. MODIFY HOW YOU PREPARE THE FOODS HE'S EATING, AND MAKE GRADUAL CHANGES.

6. DO SERVE IN COURSES, RATHER THAN HAVING ALL THE FOOD ON THE TABLE AT THE SAME TIME.

7. DON'T CORRECT HIM PUBLICLY WHEN HE'S NOT PERFECT. INSTEAD, ACKNOWLEDGE HIS SUCCESSES.

8. DO ENCOURAGE HIM TO EXERCISE.

9. DO HELP HIM PLAN FOR SOCIAL EVENTS THAT COULD CAUSE DIFFICULTY.

10. DO UNDERSTAND HOW DIFFICULT IT IS FOR HIM TO LOSE WEIGHT AND KEEP IT OFF.

1. Don't tell anyone he's trying to lose weight.

For most men, weight loss is a very private undertaking. Particularly if he's lost weight and gained it back, or has talked about wanting to lose weight and has not, he may feel sensitive about this topic. Men like to be successful, and if this is an area where they've failed, they'd rather not let anybody know. It's much better to have people come up to him and say, "Bob, you look great! How much weight have you lost?" than to have them say, "Hey, Bob, how's your diet going?" Let him take the public lead in discussing what he's doing about weight loss or how he's doing it.

2. Talk with him in a way that makes him want to listen.

Men like to be approached directly and simply. They hear messages that are both sensitive and unemotional. They reject the concept of "dieting" (which is why I don't use that word in *Lean & Mean*), but are more responsive to "getting healthy and fit." They will listen and appreciate your saying something like, "I'm concerned about your health and I think if you could lose some weight you'd feel better. What can I do to help?"

Think of yourself as a consultant or a coach. Think of your man as someone who needs essential information about his weight and health and who is currently misinformed or uninformed. When you talk with him, be specific. Talk about what food is good and why, and what food is bad and why.

But remember that ultimately he's the one who's responsible for losing weight and getting healthy, and he must decide whether or not to do anything about it.

3. Do have lots of safe foods around.

While he probably doesn't know what "safe" and "good" foods are, no doubt you do. Women have much greater access to this kind of information from their magazines and from conversations with friends. Foods that are good are "munchable," not high in fat, and thus not dangerous.

Keeping a bowl of chilled carrots, celery, or cucumbers with a very low calorie yogurt dip in the refrigerator is very useful. Also, have lots of fruit around, primarily crunchy fruit like hard green and red apples—low-calorie microwave popcorn and large pretzels. If he's an ice-cream freak, get some nonfat frozen yogurt or water-based sorbet. If you're feeling particularly domestic, put the yogurt or sorbet in cups and freeze them. Then when he goes to take some, it will be preportioned and he will be less likely to overdo it.

There are now fat-free cookies and cakes available. Substitute these for the traditional high-fat varieties. In the dairy section of grocery stores there are now a number of almost no-fat cheeses available. If cheese is "his thing," buy the no-fat kind. Having these safe foods around simply makes it easier for him to stay with his Lean & Mean Routine.

4. **Don't buy "dangerous," high-fat snacks or other foods— the kind he tends to eat when he comes home frustrated at the end of the day or while watching television in the evening or when he's working on a project late into the morning.** *Dump the junk!*

One of my first principles in helping people lose weight is to focus on environmental control—that is, not having foods in the house that are easy to abuse. So another way you can support a man's weight-loss efforts is to "dump the junk." My rule of thumb is that any snack food that has more than 20% of total calories coming from fat is dangerous and should be kept out of the house.

He may not even know what food is unhealthy and high in fat. Again, educate him. He may even think that a commercial bran muffin is healthy, but you and I know that it is a 400-calorie, sugar-laden fat sponge. He also probably doesn't know that peanuts are 180 calories an ounce with two thirds of the calories coming from fat, or that cheese is a high-fat, not a high-protein, food.

What does your man tend to eat when he is stressed or bored? Ice cream? Cheese and crackers? Chips? Candy bars? Nachos? Frozen pies or cakes? Doughnuts? Cookies? Peanut butter and jelly? Whatever it is, those are the first foods you should eliminate or substitute with no-fat alternatives. Men tend to use food (and sometimes cigarettes and alcohol) as a way of calming themselves in the face of difficult or trying situations and people. Replace the dangerous foods he usually eats with tasty, yet healthy, substitutes.

Oh, yes. Don't think that you need to keep junk food available "for the children." They will survive without it.

5. Don't serve him anything that looks or sounds like "diet food" or tiny portions. Modify how you prepare the foods he likes, and make changes gradually.

Most men have established their eating patterns fairly well by the time they're adults and will have focused on a dozen or so items that they really like. They will have also developed some attitudes about some other foods that they will consider as "suspect." For example, putting alfalfa sprouts on his salad is not likely to be well received. Ditto for tofu or spaghetti squash. If he likes ranch dressing, get a low-calorie substitute, rather than trying to shift him to oil and vinegar. If he likes red meat, reduce the frequency to only once or twice a week and buy a low-fat cut such as flank steak or top round. Prepare the meat so that it's very tasty, and serve it in multiple thin slices so it looks like a lot more. Buy a low-fat cake and serve a thin slice with a scoop of nonfat yogurt for dessert, rather than expecting him to be thrilled by a "fruit medley."

Most men are put off by very small portions, particularly at the end of the day. They often see dinner as a time to relax and "come down." As I have said previously, serve large salads, whole baked potatoes, generous servings of rice and/or pasta (with little or no fat in the sauce), so that he has a lot of food but *not* a lot of calories.

The major thrust of the Lean & Mean Program is to help men cut down the calorie density of their food, not the volume.

6. Serve meals in courses rather than family style.

Serving meals in courses means beginning with a salad, then serving an entrée, and finally offering dessert. (This, of course, doesn't mean that *you* do all the cooking, serving, and clearing. *He* can participate and so can the children.) By approaching meals in this fashion, it will prolong the amount of time that he takes to eat—which allows him to become satiated, and, thus, *reduces* the actual amount of food eaten.

Serve the way restaurants do—on plates with defined portions. Particularly if your home is one where dinner includes a lot of time for talking and kibbitzing, having additional food out of sight will greatly diminish the likelihood of his moving into unacknowledged or unthinking eating. So keep the rest of the food in the kitchen so that he has only to deal with what is put on his plate. If it's all on the table, it's just too easy to reach over and take another serving. If he wants more, have *him* go into the kitchen and get it. This, in itself, might discourage his random eating.

7. Don't correct him publicly when he's not perfect. Instead, praise him for his successes.

Think of the last time you heard someone say, "Are you sure that's on your diet?" Remember how the person being questioned looked? Think how you would feel being asked that in public— probably embarrassed.

Don't be critical or even verbally "helpful" in public. Instead, privately support every eating change he makes and heap on the praise—so long as what you're saying is truthful. As he begins to lose weight, tell him how terrific he looks. When he goes through the buffet line once (as opposed to a half dozen times, the way he used to deal with Sunday brunch), tell him later, when nobody else can hear, how great you think he handled the brunch. Let him know you noticed he only had one glass of wine at dinner, even though most of the other guests put away three or four glasses. Celebrate each ten pounds of his weight loss by doing something special together. Let him know that you know that he's doing great. As they say, "Accentuate the positive."

Other ways of supporting him positively include choosing to be with healthy, positive friends. It's useful to be around others who model healthy eating habits.

8. Do encourage him to exercise.

I believe that regular exercise is an essential part of a weight-loss and health-enhancement program. Once again, the ultimate responsibility to exercise is *his*, but there are some ways you can help. Certainly one thing you can do is join him, particularly if he's doing something like walking. Not only is he more likely to do it with you as a companion, but you can obviously benefit from this as well.

Encourage him (better yet, join him) to park your car some distance from your destination and walk to where you are going. Make an after-dinner walk a regular event in your life. The next time he asks you to go out for lunch on the weekend, suggest that you walk there instead of drive. Then take the stairs instead of the elevator. Every little step you take helps. If he wants to go to the gym, support him even if it means that you'll be having dinner a little later.

9. Do help him plan for social events that could cause difficulty.

Ingrid is a strikingly beautiful "fifty something" woman. One night I sat next to her at a banquet. When I told her I was writing this book for men, she confided to me that Jim, her husband, had become more concerned about his health in the last few years. He decided that at his age (early sixties), continuing to lose and gain weight wasn't very smart. He had made a lot of changes, but was still having a lot of trouble when they went out to dinner or to a party or to a banquet like the one we were attending.

"So what do you do?" I asked.

"Well," she said, "we talk about it before we go out to eat and I encourage Jim to plan how he's going to deal with things. We've also agreed that if it seems as though he's forgotten, it's OK for me to put my hand on his, which is our private signal that he should pay more attention to what he's eating and how much he's drinking."

"And what if he doesn't pay any attention to your signal?" I asked.

"Then he doesn't! I've done my part and the rest is up to him!"

This is a useful model to follow. If the two of you can discuss in advance how to approach the evening and if he's comfortable with your letting him know when you think there's a problem, that's a good way to go. But once again, he is ultimately responsible for how much he eats and drinks.

10. Do understand how difficult it is for him to lose the weight and keep it off.

If you also have a weight problem, then you will be immediately sympathetic. If you are either a true biological thin (your basic metabolic rate is such that you can eat fairly generous amounts of food without gaining weight), and/or you're someone who, when upset, doesn't want to eat as opposed to eating more—it may be a bit more difficult for you to understand what he's going through. But even if you do fall into one of these two categories, anything you can do that supports or encourages him to continue his efforts is in his (and your) best interests.

FINALLY

I am frequently asked by women for some guidelines about how to bring up the topic of a man's health and weight status without turning him off. They tell me that they don't understand why their attempts at being helpful sometimes backfire. Welcome to the world of gender differences!

What may be a perfectly acceptable way of talking with a woman may not be effective in talking with a man. (Books on this topic are listed in the Suggested Reading section.) So in concluding this chapter, I've chosen to focus on *how* to approach a man about his health and weight—what works, what doesn't, and why.

And by the way, no matter what technique you use, he may still choose to reject your message.

There are a whole variety of words and behaviors that *won't* work when you're trying to help a man lose weight. And there are others that *might*.

What won't work are negative or aggressive words: getting angry, "I just *hate* to see you getting so fat"; or being confrontational, "*Why* do you keep stuffing yourself?"; or insulting or judgmental, "How can you just sit there in front of the television set eating all night?" What also doesn't help is to preach or lecture.

Why? Simply because negative words often elicit the opposite reaction of what you want. Men usually react to any of the above by becoming resentful and angry themselves. They feel emasculated by your criticism. Often they become more stubborn and will reject your suggestions.

Another approach that doesn't work is nagging. While women are inclined to do what is asked of them, if it makes sense, some men are resistant to even the slightest hint that someone (and especially a woman) is trying to *tell* them what to do.

Repeating what you've just said doesn't help. Often women repeat something because they think that if he really understood what she wanted him to do, he'd do it. *Wrong!!* Usually men do hear what is being asked of them, but will intentionally wait to act on it so that they can feel they are doing it of their own free will . . . not because someone told them to do it. If a woman repeats her message again and again and again, men feel nagged at and will refuse to comply.

But don't *wait* to say anything to a man until it's too late—when he has become very overweight or has developed a serious illness. Silence is not neutral. By not saying anything, you are essentially *sanctioning* his dangerous and self-destructive behaviors.

Hinting is not effective, either. Because women have been brought up to say things indirectly, often they will hope or hint about something they want. If you soft-pedal the information you want to get to him about his health and weight, more than likely "he won't get it."

A final, nonproductive way of approaching your man is to become intensely emotional. Men report that this approach is the one that may drive them the most crazy. They have little tolerance for impassioned pleas. It makes them feel uncomfortable and irritated. Often their reaction will be to tune you out or want to get away from you.

Now let's move on to what *can* work. Men respond positively when what they hear is care or concern: "I'm *worried* that you're going to get sick." They can also be reached if you present them with a description of the situation: "I don't *know* if you have noticed, but you're eating awfully fast. How about if we both slow down and enjoy dinner?" They also respond positively to data-based information: "Just recently I *read* that even a moderate weight loss—say fifteen to twenty pounds—can have a significant impact on a man's health and will increase how long he lives."

I also find that men can respond to something when it's presented with a sense of humor. Find a *New Yorker* cartoon that makes your point. Many of the men I have worked with tell me that a good time to approach them about this subject is after dinner when the two of you are alone and he's relaxed. But do keep it to a short amount of time . . . say, a few minutes. Anything more will begin to sound like a lecture. And even though he might not respond to your efforts immediately, don't nag, but don't give up, either. Sometimes it takes a while to elicit from him the kind of positive response that you're looking for.

When you're talking to your man, use words such as *getting in shape, getting fit, getting healthy,* eating foods that are *healthy,* what foods are *good* and *bad* for you. They tend to respond less well to words like *diets, dieting, calorie counting,* or *being fat.*

Remember, *you can't do it for him.* You can prepare perfect meals, have all the right things in the house, and use all of the gender-appropriate language, but when he goes out with his colleagues, he may still choose to have two drinks before dinner, blue cheese dressing on his salad, prime rib, baked potato with butter, three glasses of wine, and mud pie for dessert. Or, he can order club soda and lime, salad with dressing on the side, broiled swordfish, and rice pilaf, drink one glass of wine, and have fresh raspberries for dessert.

It's up to him.

CHAPTER 14

THE LAST WORD

YOU'RE IN CHARGE

One of the more exciting things that's occurred in the past decade is that increasing numbers of people are coming to understand that they can influence their health status. If your father died from a heart attack at age sixty, it doesn't mean that you are destined to go the same way!

If, of course, he smoked and you smoke; if he was fifty pounds overweight and you're fifty pounds overweight; if he ate bacon and eggs for breakfast, hamburgers and fries for lunch, and pot roast and gravy for dinner and you eat the same way; if he never exercised and you never exercise; if he was a hard-driving, no-relaxation fellow and so are you—then guess what? You're on the same road that he was.

But if you don't smoke, keep your weight in a normal range, eat a low-fat diet, exercise regularly, and keep some balance between work and play, then you can live a longer and happier and healthier life. It's up to you.

COMING DOWN THE PIKE

There are some rather exciting things to look forward to. By the time this book is published, one or more pharmaceutical companies will probably have gotten FDA approval to market a new class of anti-obesity drugs that affect our brain chemistry and make it easier to adhere to a well-structured weight loss program. These drugs are useful as long as you take them, but unless you're planning to stay on them for the rest of your life, it's still up to you to learn how to manage without the pharmacological crutch.

Artificial sweeteners with no calories have been joined by synthetic fats with no calories. It would seem as though we're approaching a time when you *can* have your cake and eat it, too! However, I'm a little bit worried about people having daily hot fudge sundaes made of phony fat, phony sugar, and phony fudge—better a bit of the real thing, less frequently, than ersatz food on a regular basis.

So far as I know there are no exercise pills in the pipeline, but who can tell!

HANGING IN THERE

If you've gotten to this chapter and have actually been doing the things that I've suggested—avoiding fats, engaging in regular exercise, controlling alcohol, and not eating in response to stress—you've probably found it's not all that difficult.

But you've probably also found that you're somewhat unpredictable—some days it's easy to be in control, some days it's hard. Every once in a while you'll say, "Oh, what the hell," and order the prime rib rather than the broiled swordfish.

But you know what? That's okay. If you're following *most* of my suggestions, *most* of the time, you're already doing better than 90% of the men in this or any other developed country. You're losing weight. You're feeling better. Your cholesterol is probably lower. Your cardiovascular efficiency is increasing, your fat mass is decreasing and it'll continue to get better.

The main thing you need to do is Hang in There.

TALK TO ME

By the way, I am very interested in what you've experienced. I want to know what was helpful and really worked for you. I want to know what didn't make much sense when you tried to do it. I want to know what *you* have found successful and how you have solved certain kinds of problems so that I can share your success with other men. Please let me know by writing me at:

> Scripps Clinic and Research Foundation
> 10666 North Torrey Pines Rd.
> La Jolla, CA 92037

Remember—you don't have to be perfect—just consistent. GO FOR IT!

CALORIES AND FAT PERCENT OF COMMON FOODS

In putting together this section I consulted a variety of books, pamphlets, and government publications and information on food labels and packages. In many instances, the information that is provided is more than you could absorb, and it's presented in ways that are inconsistent and confusing. What I've done is to make things simple.

Since I recommended that animal protein be limited to 6-ounce servings, the listing of poultry, beef, pork, lamb, veal, fish, and shellfish are listed as 6-ounce servings to make comparisons easy. By the way, when you go to a restaurant, you're likely to get much more than a 6-ounce serving, so the total calories are somewhat conservative. What you should do is compare total calories and what percent of those calories come from fat.

So deciding to have a large (12 oz.) serving of well-marbled prime rib can give you an entrée of more than 1,000 calories with 60% of those calories coming from fat, while deciding to have a 6-ounce portion of broiled halibut instead will provide you with 160 calories with 10% coming from fat. The choice is yours.

In listing fruits and vegetables we are either talking about the whole fruit, i.e., *an* apple, *an* orange, *a* banana, *a* plum, or a ½-cup serving.

Cereal, grains, rice, and pasta are listed in one-cup servings. Sandwiches usually contain about 3 ounces of meat, so that's what we've listed for luncheon meats. In dealing with snacks, I've provided the portion size in which these foods are generally found—a one-ounce package of potato chips or a whole candy bar.

Using this section, I want you to become aware of the consequences of going into a party and taking a handful of popcorn (approximately 25 calories) as opposed to taking a handful of cashews (approximately 750 calories). Once you know what you're doing, the choice is yours.

By the way, the calorie and percentage of fat values are *approximate* and have been rounded off.

APPROXIMATE CALORIES AND PERCENT FAT OF COMMON FOODS

	Portion	Calories	% Fat Calories
BREADS AND SUCH			
Bagel	1 whole	200	5%
Breads (white, wheat, rye, etc.	1 slice	75	5%
Croissant	1 whole	300	50%
English muffin	1 whole	150	26%
Muffin (bran, blueberry, etc.)	1 whole	400	50%
CEREALS—COLD*			
All-Bran	1 oz.	70	6%
Cheerios	1 oz.	110	15%
Corn Chex	1 oz.	110	2%
Corn Flakes	1 oz.	110	8%
Cracklin' Oat Bran	1 oz.	110	33%
Fiber One	1 oz.	60	15%
Fruit & Fiber	1 oz.	90	10%
Granola	1 oz.	127	28%
Grape-Nuts	1 oz.	104	1%

* Almost all packaged cereals are about 100 calories an ounce, but vary considerably in terms of added sugars and amount of bran—check the labels. Brands come and go, so yours may or may not be listed. Also remember to use low-fat or nonfat milk with your cereals.

APPROXIMATE CALORIES AND PERCENT FAT
OF COMMON FOODS (*CONTINUED*)

	Portion	*Calories*	*% Fat Calories*
Shredded Wheat	1 biscuit	84	1%
Nutri-Grain, wheat	1 oz.	102	2%
Product 19	1 oz.	100	0%
Quaker 100% Natural	1 oz.	136	37%
Raisin Bran	1 oz.	120	8%
Rice Krispies	1 oz.	110	0%
Special K	1 oz.	110	0%
Total	1 oz.	110	8%
Wheaties	1 oz.	100	5%
CEREAL—HOT			
Cream of Wheat	1 cup	75	3%
Hominy grits	1 cup	85	1%
Oatmeal	1 cup	105	15%
CHEESE			
Blue—Roquefort	1 oz.	100	80%
Brie/camembert	1 oz.	90	75%
Cheddar	1 oz.	100	75%
Colby—Jack	1 oz.	110	75%
Cottage, creamed	½ cup	117	40%
Cottage, 1% fat	½ cup	82	10%
Cream cheese	1 oz.	99	90%
Jarlsberg	1 oz.	100	65%
Monterey Jack	1 oz.	110	45%
Parmesan/Romano grated	1 oz.	130	65%
Swiss	1 oz.	110	65%
CHICKEN/TURKEY*			
Light meat—no skin	6 oz.	250	25%
Dark meat—no skin	6 oz.	300	30%
Light/dark meat with skin	6 oz.	425	50%
DAIRY PRODUCTS			
Milk			
whole	1 cup	150	50%
low-fat	1 cup	120	35%

* The skin should be removed before eating chicken or turkey.

APPROXIMATE CALORIES AND PERCENT FAT
OF COMMON FOODS (CONTINUED)

	Portion	Calories	% Fat Calories
nonfat	1 cup	90	0%
Butter	1 pat	50	100%
Margarine	1 pat	50	100%
DESSERTS			
Cakes			
Angel food cake	1/12 cake	150	1%
Cheesecake	1/8 cake	225	35%
Chocolate cake	1/12 cake	300	30%
Pound cake	1/12 cake	130	50%
White cake	1/12 cake	300	30%
Ice Cream/Frozen Desserts			
Ice cream—gourmet	1/2 cup	300	70%
Ice milk—vanilla	1/2 cup	90	33%
Sherbet	1/2 cup	135	13%
Frozen yogurt			
low-fat	1/2 cup	110	10%
nonfat	1/2 cup	80	0%
Sorbet	1/2 cup	80	0%
Pastries			
Bear claw	1	250	55%
Cinnamon roll	1	250	35%
Danish	1	400	50%
Doughnuts, glazed	1	250	50%
Pies			
Apple	1/8 pie	300	40%
Cherry	1/8 pie	250	40%
Coconut cream	1/8 pie	250	60%
Lemon meringue	1/8 pie	350	35%
Pumpkin	1/8 pie	325	35%

Approximate Calories and Percent Fat of Common Foods (*Continued*)

	Portion	Calories	% Fat Calories
Fish*			
Bass	6 oz.	175	25%
Cod	6 oz.	190	10%
Flounder	6 oz.	200	10%
Halibut	6 oz.	160	10%
Mahimahi	6 oz.	150	12%
Salmon	6 oz.	300	30%
canned	6 oz.	300	35%
smoked	6 oz.	300	50%
Snapper	6 oz.	150	10%
Sole	6 oz.	125	10%
Swordfish	6 oz.	250	25%
Tuna—water packed	6½ oz.	180	20%
Fruit			
Apple	1	57	4%
Apricots	2	32	7%
Banana	1	105	2%
Blueberries	½ cup	118	2%
Cantaloupe	1 cup	57	6%
Cherries	10	49	13%
Dates—dried	½ cup	230	0%
Figs—dried	10	475	4%
Grapefruit	½ medium	39	2%
Grapes	½ cup	29	5%
Honeydew	½ cup	66	8%
Mango	1 medium	135	4%
Nectarine	1 medium	67	8%
Orange	1 medium	65	1%
Peach	1 medium	37	2%
Pear	1 medium	98	9%
Pineapple	½ cup	37	2%
Plum	1 medium	36	3%

* All values are for fresh or broiled fish.

APPROXIMATE CALORIES AND PERCENT FAT
OF COMMON FOODS (*CONTINUED*)

	Portion	Calories	% Fat Calories
Raisins	½ cup	225	0%
Strawberries	½ cup	23	4%
Tangerine	1 medium	37	2%
Watermelon	½ cup	25	4%
LUNCHEON MEATS*			
Beef, roast	3 oz.	250	45%
Bologna	3 oz.	250	75%
Chicken roll	3 oz.	90	45%
Salami	3 oz.	225	75%
Turkey Breast	3 oz.	100	25%
Turkey ham	3 oz.	100	25%
Turkey pastrami	3 oz.	100	30%
MEATS†			
Beef			
Hamburger, lean	4 oz.	300	40%
Hamburger, regular	4 oz.	400	65%
London Broil	6 oz.	300	20%
Pot roast, braised	6 oz.	400	40%
Short ribs, braised/lean	6 oz.	500	55%
Prime rib (lean and fat)	6 oz.	600	60%
Steak (porterhouse			
rib eye, T-bone, etc.)	6 oz.	400	45%
Lamb			
Leg, roasted	6 oz.	325	35%
Loin Chop, broiled	6 oz.	350	40%
Rib chop, roasted	6 oz.	400	50%
Shoulder, roasted	6 oz.	350	45%
Ribs (lean and fat)	6 oz.	600	60%

* There are low-fat varieties of many of these items now available in supermarkets. However, you're likely to get the standard variety in most restaurants.
† These calorie values and percentage fat values can vary considerably depending on the grade of meat (i.e., select, choice, or prime), how much fat remains after trimming, and how much fat is lost during the cooking process.

APPROXIMATE CALORIES AND PERCENT FAT
OF COMMON FOODS (CONTINUED)

	Portion	Calories	% Fat Calories
Pork			
Ham, fresh, roasted	6 oz.	300	40%
Ham, canned	6 oz.	225	30%
Loin, broiled	6 oz.	450	45%
Shank, roasted	6 oz.	430	45%
Spareribs, lean & fat	6 oz.	800	70%
Veal			
Steak, lean only	6 oz.	240	30%
Cutlet, lean & fat	6 oz.	360	40%
Loin chop, lean	6 oz.	400	40%
Rib, lean & fat	6 oz.	540	60%
NUTS			
Almonds	1 oz.	175	85%
Cashews	1 oz.	160	75%
Macadamia	1 oz.	200	95%
Peanuts	1 oz.	160	75%
Pecans	1 oz.	200	90%
Pistachios	1 oz.	175	80%
Walnuts	1 oz.	180	90%
PASTA AND RICE			
Pasta			
Egg noodles	1 cup	200	10%
Macaroni	1 cup	200	5%
Spaghetti	1 cup	200	5%
Rice			
Brown/white	1 cup	225	5%
Pilaf	1 cup	180	1%
Wild	1 cup	300	25%
SHELL FISH			
Clams, raw	6 oz.	100	10%
Crab, fresh	6 oz.	150	10%
Lobster	6 oz.	150	10%
Oysters, raw	6 oz.	160	20%

APPROXIMATE CALORIES AND PERCENT FAT
OF COMMON FOODS (*CONTINUED*)

	Portion	Calories	% Fat Calories
Shrimp, boiled	6 oz.	175	10%
Shrimp, fried	6 oz.	400	45%
SNACKS			
Cakes			
Crumb Cake	1	130	28%
Cupcake	1	170	32%
Ding Dongs	1	170	48%
Twinkies	1	160	28%
Candy			
Baby Ruth	1 bar	260	42%
Butterfinger	1 bar	260	42%
M&M's peanut	1 bag	240	49%
M&M's plain	1 bag	240	28%
Milk Chocolate	1 bar	254	53%
Milky Way	1 bar	290	34%
Mr. Goodbar	1 bar	296	58%
Peanut Butter cup	2 pc	280	23%
Snickers	1 bar	290	43%
Pies—snack size	1 pie	400	45%
Potato Chips/Popcorn/Pretzels			
Cheez Curls	1 oz.	160	62%
Corn Chips	1 oz.	160	56%
Popcorn, air popped	1 cup	30	3%
Popcorn, oil popped	1 cup	55	49%
Potato chips	1 oz.	160	62%
Pretzels	1 oz.	110	1%
Tortilla chips	1 oz.	140	45%
VEGETABLES			
Artichoke	1 medium	53	2%
Asparagus	½ cup	22	4%
Avocado	1 medium	300	90%

APPROXIMATE CALORIES AND PERCENT FAT
OF COMMON FOODS (CONTINUED)

	Portion	Calories	% Fat Calories
Beans			
Kidney, lima, etc.	½ cup	125	1%
Chick-peas (garbanzo)	½ cup	134	13%
Beets	½ cup	26	3%
Broccoli	½ cup	23	4%
Brussels sprouts	½ cup	30	3%
Cabbage	½ cup	10	1%
Carrot	½ cup	35	3%
Cauliflower	½ cup	15	6%
Celery	½ cup	11	8%
Collard greens	½ cup	13	7%
Corn	½ cup	89	10%
Cucumber, raw	½ cup	7	13%
Eggplant	½ cup	14	6%
Green beans	½ cup	22	4%
Lentils	½ cup	115	1%
Lettuce	½ cup	5	0%
Mushrooms	½ cup	21	4%
Onion	½ cup	29	3%
Parsley	½ cup	10	9%
Peas	½ cup	67	1%
Pepper	½ cup	18	6%
Potatoes			
Au gratin	½ cup	160	51%
Baked, w/skin, lg.	1 potato	150	0%
Boiled, small	1 potato	100	0%
French Fries	10	109	33%
Hash browns	½ cup	163	61%
Mashed	½ cup	111	32%
Scalloped	½ cup	105	43%
Radishes	½ cup	8	0%
Spinach	½ cup	21	4%

APPROXIMATE CALORIES AND PERCENT FAT
OF COMMON FOODS (*CONTINUED*)

	Portion	Calories	% Fat Calories
Squash	½ cup	50	2%
Sweet potato	½ cup	118	1%
Tomato	1 medium	24	4%
Zucchini	½ cup	9	10%
YOGURT*			
Regular plain	6 oz.	150	40%
Regular flavor/fruit	6 oz.	250	30%
Low-fat plain	6 oz.	140	25%
Low-fat flavor/fruit	6 oz.	200	20%
Nonfat plain	6 oz.	110	0%
Nonfat flavor/fruit	6 oz.	150	0%

* The calories and percentage of fat in yogurts vary enormously based upon whether they're nonfat, low-fat, or whole milk, whether they are plain or have fruit or other things added for flavor, and whether they use artificial sweetners. Read the carton.

HEALTHY RESTAURANT EATING

The average man is likely to eat as many as two or three of his meals in restaurants every day. So knowing how to act in restaurants is a key to getting and staying Lean & Mean. Restaurant eating can be pleasurable and healthy, if you follow some simple guidelines.

This appendix has been organized in the following way: First I'll give you some ideas about how to deal with restaurant breakfasts. This will be pretty simple to follow, because you'll only have to deal with one kind of food: typical American fare. Second I'll discuss different types of restaurants, giving you general guidelines for approaching all of them. Third I'll deal with the various ethnic and American restaurant menus. I'll make a series of specific recommendations regarding healthier choices, what to avoid, what to eat less frequently, and what to eat in smaller portions. Finally, I'll give you an example of a healthy meal for each kind of restaurant.

For those readers who want even more information about restaurants, I suggest that you read Nathan and Ilene Pritikin's *The Official Pritikin Guide to Restaurant Eating* and/or Hope Warshaw's *The Restaurant Companion*.

For all restaurant eating, here are some statements you can make and questions you can ask as you order your food that will help the restaurant provide you with a healthier meal:

STATEMENTS

1. "I'd like some suggestions about what to order that is low in fat."
2. "I prefer dishes that have no butter or cream."
3. "I'd like to have my meat broiled (or my fish broiled or steamed or poached)."
4. "I'd like low-fat (or nonfat) milk served with my coffee."
5. "I don't want anything that is fried."
6. "I'd like any dressing or sauce served on the side."
7. "I'd like this to be prepared with a minimum of butter, margarine, or oil."
8. "Please serve my toast (or English muffin) with butter on the side."
9. "No mayonnaise or dressing on my sandwich."
10. "I'd prefer a lean cut of meat."

QUESTIONS

1. "Is this (soup, sauce, etc.) made with cream?"
2. "Is this dish made with butter or margarine?"
3. "Can you tell me how this dish is prepared?" (i.e., fried, sautéed, etc.)
4. "Can this be made using a minimum of oil, butter or margarine?"
5. "Can you tell me what's in this dish?"
6. "Do you have any nonfat or low-fat salad dressings?"
7. "What kind of fresh vegetables do you have?"
8. "Can I have my vegetables steamed?"
9. "What kind of fresh fruit do you have?"
10. "What else would you suggest?"

BREAKFAST

Using the concept of controlling fat intake makes breakfast choices relatively easy. However, these low-fat or no-fat choices may go against what you have been eating for breakfast for many years. Therefore, my recommendation is that you eat the Lean & Mean way most of the time, but every once in a while eat what you want irrespective of how healthy it is, and have some fun.

Lean & Mean Choices	*Avoid or Limit Portion Size*
All fruit juices	Danishes
All fruit	Sweet rolls
Bagel	Sticky cinnamon rolls or buns
English muffin	Bran, blueberry, apple (or any
Hard rolls	other kind of muffins)
Toast	Doughnuts
Cold cereal (except granola)	Granola
Hot cereal	Omelettes
Poached or boiled eggs (occa-	Eggs, fried, scrambled, or Benedict
sionally)	Bacon
Egg whites anytime	Corned beef hash
Pancakes	Ham
Waffles	Steak
Low-fat or nonfat yogurt	Sausage
Canadian bacon (occasionally)	Hash brown potatoes
Jam or syrup (sparingly)	Melted butter
Corn tortilla	Coffee with half-and-half or cream
Coffee with nonfat or low-fat milk	Whole chocolate milk
Nonfat or low-fat milk	Whole milk

Remember to use only a bit of butter or margarine on your toast, bagel, English muffin, pancakes, waffles, or cereal. Use jam and syrup sparingly. Order nonfat or low-fat milk to drink or to put on cereal. If you really are in an "eggy" mood, try the following: ask the restaurant to make you a fresh (tomato and mushroom or whatever) omelet, using egg whites only, and very little butter or oil in the pan. You'll be surprised how good this will taste. Have sliced tomatoes rather than hash browns and order dry toast. You can be self-indulgent without being self-destructive.

AMERICAN RESTAURANTS

American restaurants range from national chains such as Denny's, Coco's, Bob's Big Boy, Burger King, Carl's, Houlihan's, and TGI Fridays to elegant steak and chop houses in the Midwest and East, to California-cuisine type restaurants in the West. Given the enormous range of foods that are offered at these restaurants, the best advice I can give is an overall strategy that will allow you to make good choices yet have a thoroughly enjoyable time. When eating in an American restaurant, follow these guidelines:

1. Control your portion size. European and Asian colleagues who visit the United States comment frequently on how much food we serve. Watch out for too much volume.

2. Frankly, it's often what we *add* to foods that makes them risky. While a plain hamburger with lettuce, tomato, and mustard or ketchup is a reasonable choice, make it a bacon double cheese burger and you're in Big Trouble.

3. Watch out for side dishes such as hash browns, potato salad, macaroni salad, baked potatoes topped with sour cream, cheese and bacon bits, potatoes au gratin, and "creamed" anything. Use salsa, picante sauce, or a bit of sour cream on baked potatoes, and order your vegetables steamed, without sauces.

4. Watch out for bread and rolls with lots of butter—each pat of butter or margarine is 50 calories of pure fat.

5. Also be careful with desserts. Mud pies, chocolate brownies, cheesecakes, cakes, pies, and sundaes can be an unhealthy wipeout.

Lean & Mean Choices	*Avoid or Limit Portion Size*

Appetizer/First Course

Oysters or claims on the half shell	Chicken nuggets
Shrimp cocktail	Pastas with a cream base

Lean & Mean Choices	*Avoid or Limit Portion Size*
Manhattan clam chowder	Salads with blue cheese or Roque-
Onion soup (without cheese)	fort or ranch, or Thousand Island
Green salads	dressings
Any kind of vegetable soup without	Caesar salad
a cream base	Fried cheeses
Fresh steamed vegetables	New England clam chowder
Any fruits or melons	Onion soup (with cheese)
	Soups with a cream base

MAIN COURSE/ENTRÉE

Steamed lobster (watch the butter)	Fried shrimp
Steamed crab	Chicken fried steak
Scallops	Prime rib
Broiled, steamed, or poached fish:	Spareribs
halibut, tuna, snapper, shark,	Ham
swordfish, etc.	Pork or lamb chops
Broiled chicken (remove the skin)	Any meats served with gravies
Game hen (remove the skin)	Hamburgers
Turkey (remove the skin)	Hot dogs
Filet mignon (small)	Fried meats including liver and on-
Pastas with tomato sauce	ions, chicken or veal cutlet
Any rice, bean, or legume dishes	Roast beef, pork, or lamb
(ask about how it is prepared)	Sausages
	Most stews
	Most casseroles
	Pastas with meat or cream sauce

DESSERT

Angel food cake	Pies (especially à la mode)
Fresh	Cakes (except angel food)

Lean & Mean Choices	*Avoid or Limit Portion Size*
Frozen yogurt	Cheesecake
Sorbet	Ice cream sundaes
	Ice cream
	Puddings

Example of a healthy meal:

1. Appetizer—shrimp cocktail
2. First course—green salad, dressing on the side
3. Main course—broiled halibut, baked potato with salsa, picante sauce, or a bit of sour cream
4. Dessert—sorbet, fresh fruit

Example of a meal to avoid:

1. Appetizer—fried zucchini
2. First course—salad with blue cheese dressing
3. Main course—barbeque spare ribs, creamy cole slaw and baked beans
4. Dessert—mud pie

CHINESE RESTAURANTS

Chinese restaurants can be wonderful places to eat, but you do need to exert some control. Cantonese restaurants tend to be safer than either Mandarin, Szechuan, or Hunan, because Cantonese food is characterized by stir-fry wok cooking, and stir-fried food tends to have less fat. When eating in a Chinese restaurant, follow these guidelines:

1. Avoid fried rice, fried noodles, or crispy noodles. These tend to be fat laden.

2. Concentrate on rice and vegetable dishes or vegetable dishes mixed with small amounts of meat, poultry, fish, or shell fish.

3. Ask your waiter to have your food prepared by steaming it, or using

chicken stock as a base for stir-fry. If there is resistance, ask him or her to use *very little oil* in food preparation. Also ask that food be served without MSG.

4. Have your meal service slowed down so that you have an opportunity to eat leisurely and become satiated. Order extra rice and put other food on top of it, rather than using rice as the accompaniment to the food.

5. Use chopsticks and drink lots of tea.

Lean & Mean Choices	*Avoid or Limit Portion Size*

APPETIZER/FIRST COURSE

Soups of all kinds:	Egg rolls
Egg flower	Spring rolls
Wonton	Fried shrimp
Wor wonton	Barbecued spareribs
Sizzling rice	Fried wonton
Hot and sour	Gotlet chicken
Seaweed	Rumaki
Steamed Dim sum (with vegetable or seafood filling)	Crispy noodles

MAIN COURSE/ENTRÉE

Shrimp with lobster sauce	Sweet and sour shrimp, chicken, or pork
Cashew shrimp	Shrimp fried rice
Kung Pao shrimp	Chicken fried rice
Shrimp with mixed vegetables	Barbecue pork fried rice
Any steamed, broiled or poached fish	Fried rice
Almond chicken	Ginger beef
Cashew chicken	Curried beef with tomato

Lean & Mean Choices	*Avoid or Limit Portion Size*
Chicken or vegetable chop suey	Mongolian beef
Chicken with water chestnut and snow peas	Beef with oyster sauce
	Peking duck
Kung Pao chicken	Duck of any kind
Chicken with mixed vegetables	Any pork dishes
Beef with mixed vegetables (small portion)	Pepper steak
Egg fu yung (small portion)	
Vegetable, chicken or shrimp chow mein	
Steamed or simmered tofu (in small amounts)	
White rice	

DESSERT

Fortune cookie	Almond cookies
Fruit	Ice cream

An example of how to order in a Chinese restaurant for four people:

1. Appetizer—bowl of Wor Wonton soup
2. Main Courses—a double order of white rice and dishes that would include Kung Pao shrimp, chicken with water chestnuts and snow peas, mixed vegetables, and vegetarian chow mein
3. Dessert—Fortune cookie

An example of a meal to avoid:

1. Appetizer—Egg rolls
2. Main courses—B.B.Q. Spare Ribs, Fried rice, Mongolian beef, egg

fu yung, Sweet and sour shrimp and pork chow mein with fried noodles
3. Dessert—almond cookies

FRENCH RESTAURANTS

I love going to French restaurants, because the food is usually prepared with care and presented in a way that is appealing to the eye as well as the palate. By the same token, French restaurants can be dangerous because traditional French cooking emphasizes butter and cream-based sauces, entrées that are sautéed (panfried), and rich desserts. However, things are changing. Recently, there has been a movement toward "nouvelle cuisine," which attempts to maintain most of the flavor (and the sensations) of traditional French cooking without the heavy butter/cream-based sauces. When eating in a French restaurant, follow these guidelines:

1. Avoid or only taste traditionally high-fat appetizers such as pâté or escargot. They are simply loaded with fat.
2. Watch out for the sauces—béarnaise, hollandaise, béchamel, Mornay, beurre-anything, meunière, Crème Fraiche, etc. Avoid them entirely or have them "on-the-side."
3. Choose entrées carefully. Watch out for duck (unless the skin has been removed) or large servings of beef, lamb or veal—particularly when heavily sauced. Focus more on fish, shellfish, or poultry entrées.
4. Order à la carte items rather than prix fixe meal. You'll have less food to deal with.
5. Be wary of the desserts. If you are going to get a traditional dessert, split it at least two (if not more) ways. If not, order sorbet or a fresh fruit selection.

Lean & Mean Choices	*Avoid or Limit Portion Size*

Appetizer/First Course

Clams and oysters on the half shell	Sautéed shrimp
Steamed mussels and clams	Escargot
Shrimp cocktail	Marinated artichoke hearts
Caviar	Cheeses
Steamed vegetables	Creamed soups of any kind includ-
Cold asparagus or other vegetables	ing vegetables
House salad	Bisques
Bouillons	Pâtés and terrines
Consommés	Onion soup (with cheese)
Onion soup (without cheese)	Omelettes
Aspic (with no cream)	

Main Course/Entrée

Shell Fish	Lobster with butter
Fish grilled, poached, or boiled	Lobster thermidor
Fish in wine sauce (or sauce on the	Fish in cream sauce
side), including salmon, sole,	Any fish, poultry or meat that is
tuna, halibut, swordfish, etc.	sautéed, fricasseed, or stewed
Bouillabaisse	Chicken in cream or cheese sauce
Poultry in wine sauce (with no	Chicken Wellington
cream)	Duck à l'orange
Poultry in mustard sauce (with no	Fricasseed chicken
cream)	Goose
Coq au vin	T-bone or porterhouse steak
Breast of duck (with skin removed)	Beef en croûte
Filet mignon (small serving)	
Tournedos of beef (sauce on the	
side)	

Lean & Mean Choices	Avoid or Limit Portion Size
Medallions of veal or lamb (sauce on the side) Beef Bourguignonne (small portion) Bouillabaisse	Veal Oscar Any meats or poultry w/stuffing or meat or vegetable Cheese quiche Gratin (casseroles w/cheese) Crepe with cream sauce Cassoulet Soufflé Fondue

DESSERT

Meringue Sorbet Fresh raspberries Fresh strawberries Fresh melon	Soufflé Custard Crepes Ice cream Sundae Cheese platter Chocolate fondue Crème caramel Mousse Baba and Savarin Tart

Example of a healthy meal:

1. Appetizer—Steamed mussels in a white wine sauce
2. Second course—Asparagus with a vinaigrette sauce on the side
3. Main course—Coq au vin (just check to see that scant butter or margarine is used in the preparation), new potatoes
4. Dessert—Raspberry sorbet

Example of a meal to avoid:

1. Appetizer—Pâté
2. First Course—Salad with Roquefort dressing
3. Main course—Beef en croûte, Lyonnaise potatoes
4. Dessert—Napoleon

ITALIAN RESTAURANTS

The kinds of Italian restaurants that one might go to range from a neighborhood pizzeria to a more elegant Northern Italian restaurant that emphasizes fish, chicken, beef, or veal dishes. When you think of Italian food, what's the first thing that comes to mind? Pasta. All pasta, no matter what shape, is a healthy food. Broad noodles are used in lasagna, while angel hair pasta, regular spaghetti, or linguini are usually served with sauces. The problem is not with the pasta, but what's on top of it, layered between it, or what it's covered with. Many pastas, such as cappelletti, ravioli, and tortellini, are filled with cheese or high-fat meats and must be eaten sparingly. If you want to eat pizza, order the vegetarian variety (without black olives) and limit yourself to two slices. If you want to be really healthy, ask the restaurant to prepare it *without* cheese. When eating in an Italian restaurant, follow these guidelines:

1. If at all possible, order foods that are vegetable- and pasta-based as opposed to meat- and cheese-based.
2. Ask lots of questions about how sauces are prepared and whether they can be served on the side.
3. Watch out for food such as garlic bread, which tends to contain a lot of butter or oil.
4. Share an entrée or order an appetizer as an entrée.
5. If you are going to have a traditional dessert, share it.

Lean & Mean Choices   *Avoid or Limit Portion Size*

APPETIZER/FIRST COURSE

Clams on the half shell
Oysters on the half shell
Steamed clams
Steamed mussels
Clams or mussels in a tomato sauce
Minestrone soup
Pasta e fagioli soup (beans and
  pasta)
Other vegetable based soups
Consommé
Steamed vegetables (sauce on the
  side)
Cervichi
Steamed calamari with tomato sauce
House salad

Antipasto
Roasted peppers in oil
Fried calamari
Fried zucchini or other vegetables
Clams casino
Frittata
Sausage
Salami
Meat- or cream-based soups
Spinach salad
Caesar salad

Lean & Mean Choices   *Avoid or Limit Portion Size*

MAIN COURSE/ENTRÉE

Fish—any of the following:
  poached, broiled, or baked (or
  with sauces on the side) bass,
  halibut, sole, snapper, shrimp,
  scampi, squid, etc.
Breast of chicken
Chicken cacciatore
Broiled chicken
Chicken piccata (very little butter)
Polenta
Sirloin steak (small)
Medallions of beef (small serving)
Medallions of lamb (small serving)

Fish prepared in cream or white
  sauces (such as alfredo)
Fried chicken
Chicken parmigiana
Chicken w/mushrooms & arti-
  chokes
Chicken with sausage
Veal parmigiana
Vitello tonnato (veal in cream
  sauce)
Veal parmigiana
Veal w/pesto and mozzarella cheese
Breaded veal cutlet

Lean & Mean Choices

Veal piccata (little butter)
Broiled veal chop (small, lean)
All pastas (Fettuccine, penne, ver-
    micelli, spaghetti with tomato-
    based sauce)
Vegetarian lasagna ($1/2$ portion,
    without cheese)
Vegetarian pizza (2 slices)

Avoid or Limit Portion Size

Stuffed veal cutlet
Any pastas w/cream-based sauce or
    meat, or stuffing (fettuccini al-
    fredo, cannelloni)
Vitello tonnato (veal in cream
    sauce)
Eggplant parmigiana
Meat lasagna & ravioli
Pizza with sausage, pepperoni

DESSERT

Fresh raspberries
Strawberries
Blueberries
Fresh melon
Sorbet
Meringue

Zabaglione
Rum cake
Cheese cake
Ice cream, tortoni, gelato, tartufa
Cream caramel
Flan
Torta
Rice pudding
Strudel
Mascarpone

Example of a healthy meal:

1. Appetizer—Steamed clams
2. First course—Minestrone soup
3. Main course—Broiled halibut with a side of angel hair pasta with
   marinara sauce
4. Dessert—Raspberry sorbet

Example of a meal to avoid:

1. Appetizer—Fetuccini alfredo
2. First course—Caesar salad

3. Main course—Veal parmigiana with a side of fried zucchini

4. Dessert—cheese cake

JAPANESE RESTAURANTS

The main problem with eating in a Japanese restaurant has little to do with fat and a lot to do with sodium. If you are on a salt-restricted diet and/or have high blood pressure, you may need to limit the frequency with which you visit Japanese restaurants. Consult with your physician and/or a registered dietitian if you need more information.

Aside from that, Japanese restaurants are a wonderful place to eat, because food is prepared simply, meat and fish are often used as accompaniment rather than a major part of the meal, and rice and noodles are served in abundance. Most of all, Japanese food looks, smells, and tastes terrific.

By the way, traditional Japanese restaurants are not the same as Japanese steak houses.

When eating in a Japanese restaurant, follow these guidelines:

1. If you have concerns about sodium, use very little of the dipping sauces that accompany the food.

2. Focus on fish items. And if you have a yen for raw fish, sashimi and sushi are your choices.

3. Order an extra pot of rice for the table. In most Japanese restaurants, fried rice is not even an alternative.

4. The only fried food that is usually served in a Japanese restaurant is tempura. Eat it less often and/or in smaller portions.

5. One-pot entrées that are cooked or heated at the table such as Yosenabe (a fish, chicken, and noodle stew) or Shabu shabu (a variant, containing shell fish) are wonderful choices.

| *Lean & Mean Choices* | *Avoid or Limit Portion Size* |

APPETIZER/FIRST COURSE

Green salad	Tempura of any kind
Miso soup	
Assorted sushi	
Assorted sashimi	

MAIN COURSE/ENTRÉE

Sukiaki (beef with vegetables and noodles in a broth, often cooked at your table)	Pork cutlet
	Kobe beef
	Tempura of any kind
Shabu shabu (thinly sliced beef & vegetables cooked at your table)	
Sushi and sashimi	
Yose-nabe (shrimp, mussels, fish, chicken, and vegetables in a special broth, cooked at your table)	
Chicken teriyaki	
Chicken yakitori	
Beef teriyaki	
White and brown rice	

DESSERT

Fresh fruit	Ice cream

Example of a healthy meal:

1. Appetizer—Salad, miso soup, or assorted sushi
2. Main course—Yose-nabe (shared with others), white rice
3. Dessert—Fresh fruit

Example of a meal to avoid:

1. Appetizer—Tempura
2. Main course—Pork cutlet or Kobe beef
3. Dessert—Ice cream

JEWISH DELICATESSENS

Having spent the early years of my life in Brooklyn and being the son of eastern European Jewish immigrants, I would love to be able to tell you that traditional Jewish cooking is hearty, nutritious, delicious, and healthy. But I can't. Unfortunately, while it is hearty and delicious, healthy and nutritious it's not. But there are ways to deal appropriately with this type of food.

The secret is to control portion size and to be very selective about what it is you order. In general, you will need to avoid most of the traditional appetizers and focus more on dishes that are more simply prepared. Sandwiches tend to be a staple in delicatessens, so I'm listing these as main courses. Most restaurants will serve these in portions that are ample—too ample, in fact. So ordering a half of a sandwich will usually suffice. I'll also be describing traditional entrées, since there are some that you can eat with relative comfort, so long as you don't do it too often.

When eating in a Jewish restaurant/delicatessen, follow these guidelines:

1. Many of the traditional entrées from eastern European origins are loaded with fat. If you don't know what is contained in the food, ask the waiter/waitress. You'll generally get more information than you bargain for.

2. Watch out for foods such as Russian dressing (Thousand Island), coleslaw (which is mayonnaise-based), or potato salad (which is also filled with mayonnaise). Eating these will compromise an otherwise reasonable meal.

3. If you are at all salt sensitive, watch out for sauerkraut and/or pickles, which are sometimes served in a "help-yourself" manner. While calories are low, sodium content is very high.

4. If you are going to have a delicatessen sandwich, use the words "lean" and "well trimmed" and look the waiter or waitress right in his or her eye. Avoid having cheese on the sandwich or ordering "combination" sandwiches.

5. Watch out for the desserts such as cheese cake, strudel, and Danishes. Eat them rarely. Or if you want some, share it with your eating companion.

Lean & Mean Choices   *Avoid or Limit Portion Size*

APPETIZER/FIRST COURSE

Green salad (dressing on the side)   Chicken soup with kreplach
Matzo ball soup   Chopped chicken liver
Chicken soup with noodles   Creamed herring
Chicken soup with rice   Noodle kugel
Gefilte fish
Beef borscht
Cabbage borscht
Herring in wine sauce

MAIN COURSE/ENTRÉE

Broiled fish   Blintzes
Roast turkey   Latkes (fried potato pancakes)
Roast chicken   Grilled knockwurst
Chicken in the pot   Kishke (stuffed derma)
Turkey sandwich (no mayonnaise)   Kreplach (Jewish ravioli)
Tongue sandwich   Combination sandwiches, e.g.,
Corned beef sandwich—lean ($^1/_2$)   corned beef/Swiss cheese,
Pastrami sandwich—lean ($^1/_2$)   coleslaw and Russian dressing
Roast beef sandwich—lean ($^1/_2$)   Liverwurst sandwich
                                         Bagel, lox, and cream cheese
                                         Short ribs

Lean & Mean Choices	_Avoid or Limit Portion Size_

DESSERT

Fruit compote	Cheesecake
Fresh melon	Strudel
Fresh berries of any kind (blueberries, raspberries, strawberries)	Cream pie
	Cake

Example of a healthy meal:

1. Appetizer—Matzo ball soup
2. First course—Green salad, dressing on the side
3. Main course—Roast chicken (remove the skin), roasted potatoes
4. Dessert—Fruit compote

Example of a meal to avoid:

1. Appetizer—Chopped chicken liver
2. First course—Chicken soup with kreplach
3. Main course—Braised short ribs with potato pancakes
4. Dessert—Chocolate cheese cake

MEXICAN RESTAURANTS

Mexican restaurants and their close cousin, Southwestern restaurants, have become quite popular in the last few years. Basic Mexican food with its emphases on rice, corn tortillas and cooked beans, chili and salsa are terrific, healthy foods. However, change the corn tortillas to flour, add a heavy cheese sauce, stuff the tortillas with beef, refry the beans, and serve this with side orders of guacamole, sour cream and black olives and you're in Big Trouble. However, with a little bit of planning and following some basic rules, dining in Mexican and Southwestern restaurants can be a tasty and healthy experience. When eating in a Mexican restaurant, follow these guidelines:

1. Use salsa as your primary flavoring agent, since it is very low calorie and fat free. Whenever possible, order corn tortillas, not flour. Corn tortillas are made from corn flour mixed with water and lime, whereas flour tortillas are made with flour and lard.

2. Watch out for the basket of corn chips—they're likely to be fried. Take only a few and dip them in salsa, not guacamole.

3. Watch out for the beans. Refried means that they have been mixed with lard. If they are cooked in any other manner, they are likely to be a good alternative.

4. When possible, substitute fish or poultry for high-fat meat fillings (e.g., chicken burrito as opposed to beef burrito, fish taco rather than pork taco), and order single items rather than combination plates.

5. Always ask to have the guacamole and/or sour cream either eliminated or significantly reduced. If it's on your plate, you are more likely to eat it. If it's not, you're not likely to miss it.

Lean & Mean Choices	*Avoid or Limit Portion Size*

APPETIZER/FIRST COURSE

Lean & Mean Choices	Avoid or Limit Portion Size
Salad with dressing on the side (use salsa as your main dressing)	Chimichangas
	Chips and guacamole
Spicy cold vegetables with salsa	Nachos (chips w/melted cheese)
Vegetarian chili	Chili con carne
Black bean soup	Quesadillas (tortillas with melted cheese)
Gazpacho	
Corn tortillas with salsa	
Seviche	

Lean & Mean Choices	*Avoid or Limit Portion Size*

MAIN COURSE/ENTRÉE

Shrimp (carmarines)	Eggs (huevos)
Fish with rice or beans	Super nachos
Chili	Chile rellano
Chicken or shrimp fajitas or burritos (grilled, if possible with no sour cream and guacamole)	Beef burrito
	Beef taco
	Beef enchiladas (w/melted cheese)
Chicken tostada (no guacamole, on a corn tortilla)	Beef fajitas
	Beef quesadillas
Chicken enchilada (light or no cheese)	Chorizo
	Mexican steak
Grilled chicken, fish, or shrimp	Flautas
Chicken taco (minimal cheese, soft corn tortilla)	Chicken Mole
	Carne Asada
Chicken tamale (light or no cheese)	Chile con queso
Taco chicken salad	Fried tortillas
Black beans	Chile rellano
Mexican rice (arroz)	
Red and green salsa	

DESSERT

Fruit	Ice cream
Sorbet	Pastries
	Flan
	Sopaipillas

Example of a healthy meal:

1. Appetizer—Cold vegetables and salsa
2. First course—Black bean soup

   3. Main course—Chicken fajitas, side of rice
   4. Dessert—Sorbet

Example of a meal to avoid:

   1. Appetizer—Chips and guacamole
   2. First course—Quesadillas
   3. Main course—Chile rellano with refried beans
   4. Dessert—Ice cream sundae with sopaipillas

APPENDIX III

FAST FOOD CHOICES

Fast food restaurants have become a part of the American scene, and it is unusual to be in any community in which there are not at least a half dozen such establishments. Now, the problems with "fast food" restaurants are twofold. First, there is a concept of *fast*, which means that people tend to zoom in and out, grab what's handy, and often eat without thinking. A second problem is the food itself. While a number of fast food chains have recently made significant strides by offering low-fat alternatives, by and large, fast food restaurants are still high-fat, high-sodium, and high-cholesterol havens. A meal that consists of a cheese burger, a large order of French fries, large milk shake, and a chocolate chip cookie *can easily exceed 2,000 calories with more than 50% of those calorie coming from fat.*

The variety of fast food restaurants has increased dramatically over the last ten years. The burger world (McDonald's, Burger King, Jack in the Box) has now been joined by take-out pizza restaurants (Pizza Hut, Little Caesar, Domino's), and now we have emerging Mexican restaurants (Taco Bell, Del Taco, etc.). For those who want an in-depth look at fast food restaurants I strongly recommend the second edition of the *Completely Revised and Updated Fast Food Guide* by Michael F. Jacobson, Ph.D., and Sarah Fritschner. In this appendix, I've tried to give the reader an overview of what is currently available so that he can make wise choices. Breakfast selections would best be limited to juice, plain English muffin, or a reduced-fat bran muffin, cereal with low-fat milk, or pancakes. For lunch and dinner, the best choices would be a small, plain hamburger or a broiled chicken sandwich, with a garden salad on the side, a seafood or chicken salad with reduced or no calorie dressing, and a low-fat yogurt for dessert.

Approximate Calories and Percent Fat of Usual Fast Food Items

	Calories	% Fat Calories
Beef		
Sandwiches		
Roast beef	550	50%
Bacon beef & Cheese	550	55%
Hamburger	350	40%
Bacon cheese burger	600	60%
Breakfast		
Bacon—2 slices	75	75%
Biscuits—bacon, ham, sausage	350	50%
Burritos	400	55%
Cereal with 1% milk	*160*	*10%**
Croissants—plain	200	50%
Croissants—eggs & meat	400	60%
Danish	400	50%
Muffin, regular	350	45%
English muffin	150	30%
Pancakes (3)	600	30%
Burritos		
Beef	500	40%
Bean	450	30%
Chicken	350	35%
Tacos		
Chicken	200	40%
Beef	250	50%
Dessert		
Cheese cake	300	70%
Cookie—chocolate chip	350	45%

APPROXIMATE CALORIES AND PERCENT FAT
OF USUAL FAST FOOD ITEMS (CONTINUED)

	Calories	% Fat Calories
Pie/turnover	300	45%
Shake/malt (regular)	400	30%
Shake/malt (low fat)	300	10%
Frozen yogurt—low fat	100	10%
CHICKEN		
Sandwiches		
Baked	400	35%
Broiled	300	30%
Club	550	50%
Fried	700	50%
Pieces/Parts		
Nuggets (6)	275	55%
Breast—fried (1)	400	50%
Drumstick—fried (1)	150	50%
Thigh—fried (1)	300	60%
Wing—fried (1)	200	60%
FISH		
Baked fillets	400	40%
Fried fillets	600	50%
Sandwiches	350	45%
Shrimp—fried (6)	400	60%
PIZZA—2 slices		
Cheese	400	30%
Pepperoni/sausage	500	45%
Veggie	350	30%
SALADS (without dressing)		
Chef	300	50%
Chicken	200	25%
Garden	50	25%
Seafood	200	20%
Taco with shell	900	60%
Taco without shell	500	50%

APPROXIMATE CALORIES AND PERCENT FAT OF USUAL FAST FOOD ITEMS (*CONTINUED*)

	Calories	% Fat Calories
Salad Dressing—2 oz. regular	300	75%
Salad Dressing—2 oz. low-fat	*100*	*30%*
SIDE ORDERS		
Baked potato—plain	*250*	*0%*
Baked potato—sour cream	400	30%
Baked potato—cheese	500	40%
Coleslaw (creamy)	100	50%
French fries—medium	300	50%
Mashed potato w/gravy	*75*	*20%*
Onion rings (fried—med)	400	55%

* Items in italics represent lowest calorie/percent fat choices.

Suggested Reading

DIET, EXERCISE, STRESS, AND LIFESTYLES

Bailey, Covert. *The New Fit or Fat*. Boston, Massachusetts: Houghton Mifflin, 1991.

Benson, Herbert. *The Relaxation Responses*. New York, New York: Avon Books, 1975.

Bricklin, Mark and Maggie Spilner. *Walking for Health*. Emmaus, Pennsylvania: Rodale Press, 1992.

Cooper, Kenneth H. *The New Aerobics*. New York, New York: Bantam Books, 1990.

Craig, Jenny. *What Have You Got To Lose*. New York, New York: Villard Books, 1992.

Ferguson, James. *Habits, Not Diets*. Palo Alto, California: Bull Press, 1987.

Tabias, Maine and John P. Sullivan. *Complete Stretching*. New York, New York: Alfred A. Knopf, 1992.

Weider, Joe. *Joe Weider's Ultimate Body Building*. Chicago, Illinois: Contemporary Books, 1989.

HEALTHY EATING

Debakey, Michael E. *The Living Heart Diet*. New York, New York: Simon and Schuster, 1984.

Jones, Jeanne. *Eating Smart*. New York, New York: Macmillan Publishing Co., 1990.

Ornish, Dean. *Reversing Heart Disease*. New York, New York: Random House Publishing, 1990.

Saltman, Paul and Joel Gurin and Ira Mothner. *The California Nutrition Book*. Boston, Massachusetts: Little, Brown and Company, 1987.

FOOD VALUES AND RESTAURANT GUIDES

Dennington, Jean A.T. *Food Values*. New York, New York: Harper & Row, 1989.

Jacobson, Michael F. and Sarah Fritschner. *The Completely Revised and Updated Fast Food Guide*. New York, New York: Workman, 1991.

Pritikin, Nathan and Irene Pritikin. *The Official Guide to Restaurant Eating*. New York, New York: Merrill Company, Inc., 1984.

Sonberg, Lynn. *The Quick and Easy Fat Gram and Calorie Counter*. New York, New York: Avon Books, 1992.

Warshaw, Hope S., M.M.Sc., R.D. *The Restaurant Companion*. Chicago, Illinois: Surrey Books, 1990.

MEN, WOMEN, AND COMMUNICATION

Evan Weiss, Daniel. *The Great Divide. How Men and Women Really Differ*. New York, New York: Poseidon Press, 1991.

Farrel, Warren. *Why Men Are the Way They Are*. New York, New York: McGraw-Hill, 1986.

Goldberg, Herb. *What Men Really Want*. New York, New York: Signet Books, 1991.

Shaevitz, Morton H. with Marjorie Hansen Shaevitz. *Sexual Static: How Men Are Confusing the Women They Love*. Boston, Massachusetts: Little, Brown and Co., 1988.

Tannen, Deborah. *You Just Don't Understand: Women and Men in Conversation*. New York: William Morrow Company, 1990.